EVIL MEDICINE:

Bubble, Bubble, Toil And Trouble!

by Richard Dennis

Cover designed by Peter Giordano

Disclaimer

The author is a reporter, not a doctor. These facts and opinions are expressed under the First Amendment of the US Constitution, granting the right to discuss openly and freely all matters of public concern, and to express viewpoints, no matter how controversial or unaccepted they are.

Certain persons considered experts may disagree with certain statements here. This information is for educational use only. You should not use it in any way, shape or manner as a substitute for your personal physician.

This book is dedicated to Garth.
You are an inspiration to me.

> **"We sometimes joke that when you're doing a clinical trial, there are two possible disasters. The first disaster is if you kill people. The second disaster is if you cure them. The truly good drugs are the ones you can use chronically for a long, long time.'**
> - from an anonymous biotech analyst

EVIL MEDICINE:
Bubble, Bubble, Toil And Trouble!

Table of Contents

Introduction:
"Where is Clint Eastwood When You Need Him?"

When I was in college in the 1960s, the "spaghetti westerns" (set in the US west, but made in Italy) came out. Clint Eastwood starred in several.

In one movie, Clint rode into town and found everyone terrified because some gang was coming to get revenge on the town and would probably kill every last citizen. No one, not the sheriff or any other citizen, was willing to stand up to the bad guys. They were convinced it was certain death.

So Clint took over. He used his wits and prepared the town for the inevitable onslaught. And when the gang came – probably 30 of them – they had to divide up, because of the way Clint set up the town. And he used that advantage to conquer them individually.

Clint Eastwood saved the day.

But now, the outlaws are back. Today, the gang has already ridden into town and taken over. They have more money than God. Worse, they think they ARE God! They laugh at the law. They fear no one. They leave a trail of death & destruction. And these outlaws dress in suits, or they wear stethoscopes.

But these days, Clint Eastwood is an old man. He can't help you. If you and your family are going to survive, you're going to have to help yourself.

From the Wall Street Journal June 22 2001

"In 1999, the Center for Disease Control and Prevention reported more then 600,000 hospital admissions and 700,000 emergency-room visits resulting from medications that were correctly administered but nonetheless produced side effects - from intestinal bleeding to seizures to even death."

Richard Dennis
Monticello, Florida
December, 2005

2 - The Problem In a Nutshell

Merck & Co. is a pharmaceutical giant that makes many prescription drugs. Some of their best-sellers are the statin drugs prescribed in cases of high cholesterol. Merck knows very well that statin drugs deplete your body of Coenzyme Q-10, a nutrient needed for proper muscle function (especially your heart muscle). That's why, in 1990, Merck got Patents No. 4929437 and 4933165, which combine CoQ10 with a statin drug.

But Merck never actually marketed any product from those patents.

The years have shown us that statin drugs cause widespread muscle damage, soreness & pain. If you take statins over time – and many doctors tell patients to continue the drug for the rest of their life, to keep the cholesterol level down – your muscle tissue degradation may lead to kidney damage and eventually death by toxic kidney overload. In any event, every pill you take increases your CoQ10 deficiency, harming your heart. And no place does Merck suggest you supplement with CoQ10, even though they have known it was crucial at least since 1990.

Merck's unused patents beg some questions. Like:

1. Why not add some CoQ10 to stop the pain and muscle degeneration you get with statins?

2. Is Merck worried that relieving pain with CoQ10 might affect sales of the painkillers that earn them $Billions a year?

3. Why doesn't Merck at least advise customers that they should add CoQ10 to their regimen?

4. Why don't doctors advise their statin drug patients to supplement CoQ10? Does your doctor even know the situation? Does he care?

5. Why are there no FDA rules to inform patients to add CoQ10 to their statin prescription? (Statin drugs in Canada carry the information about CoQ10.)

6. Again, it's been known for a long time that statin drugs deplete CoQ10. And yet, have you ever seen an article in any magazine or medical journal suggesting that you supplement this nutrient? They ALL carry a ton of pharmaceutical ads. Could they possibly not know? Could it be something else?

7. Knowing all this, how can any person in their right mind trust their family's health to drug companies like Merck or government agencies like the FDA, or doctors who often know nothing about nutrition?

Look. The purpose of this book is not to rip the drug companies, the FDA, the doctors, or the media. They are what they are.

The purpose of this book is to alert YOU to the fact that if you hand over responsibility for your health and your family's health to someone else, you are making an error, with the likelihood of serious consequences. If you trust the drug companies, the FDA, the doctors, the universities, and the media, then you and your family increase your risks of deteriorating health and early death.

In *"Evil Medicine,"* you will get a lot of explanation and a lot of examples of why you probably ought to think twice before you trust the "experts." And, in my opinion, it's a waste of time to try to change our current system. Too big, too engrained, and it would take way too much money to ever battle it and change it. **The only sane action is to take responsibility for your own health and your family's health. THAT is my message.**

3 – 1992: It Started With AIDS

Remember the hubbub in the late 1980s and early 1990s? AIDS was spreading, and activists across the U.S. were clamoring for chemical solutions. They were especially upset that the Food & Drug Administration approval process for new drugs took so long. Two and a half years for approval was average. Many drugs – especially those offering hope for AIDS patients – seemed to take forever.

. The activists had total drug company support in the desire to get new drugs to market faster. Together, they pressured the politicians. In 1992 Congress passed a law creating the PDUFA, the Prescription Drug User Fee Act, by which drug companies pay money to the FDA to expedite review & approval of new drugs. Under this "pay-for-play" system, drug approval time dropped to 12 months on average.

Drug companies were thrilled and came up with a raft of new drugs. It probably seemed to some that having the drug companies pay the FDA (their regulators!) for faster approval … well, it could certainly be a conflict of interest.

It Was Obvious Which Way The Political Winds Were Blowing

For the drug companies, one day's delay in a new drug hitting the market cost $1 to $2 million in profit. The drug companies actually hired crews of people to "hang out" at the FDA and do everything possible to expedite approval of new drugs.

Very few people ever voiced their misgivings about the arrangement.

So was there universal euphoria due to all the new life-saving drugs being approved by the FDA?

Hardly. According to FDA employee Dr. David Graham:

"Industry is saying there are all these lifesaving drugs that the FDA is slow to approve and people are dying in the streets because of it. The fact is that probably about two-thirds to three-quarters of the drugs that the FDA reviews are already on the market and are being reviewed for another indication.

"A very small proportion of drugs represent a new drug that hasn't been marketed before. Most of those drugs are no better than the ones that exist. If you want to talk about breakthrough drugs -- the ones that really make a difference in patients' lives and represent a revolution in pharmacology -- we're talking about maybe one or two drugs a year. Most of them aren't breakthroughs and most of them aren't life-saving, but they get treated as if they were."[1]

But the drug companies got what they wanted – fast approval for all the mass-market, high-profit drugs they could produce, to address every real and made-up awful medical condition they could manufacture.

Footnote:
1 - Graham

4 - The Chinese Finger Prison

When I was a kid, we had the Chinese finger prison. It was a small cylinder made of woven straw, with each end open. You get someone to stick their left forefinger in one end, right forefinger in the other. And he can't get out.

He pulls his fingers. The cylinder lengthens and narrows. It grabs his fingers tighter. No matter how strong he is, he can't get out pulling his fingers apart.

He finally figures out he has to push his fingers in the cylinder. This shortens the cylinder. The diameter gets bigger. His fingers come out.

If you're working on a problem, and you don't understand the nature of the problem, you make things worse. This is an important lesson to remember as we talk about all the players and events in the prescription drug fiasco.

5 – 1997: "The Perfect Storm!"

Several years ago, there was a best-selling book & movie titled, *"The Perfect Storm."* The story was based on true events from a few years prior, when two huge weather systems converged over the North Atlantic in some prime fishing ground, creating a monster killer storm.

In 1997, we saw a similar convergence in the pharmaceutical arena … with similar results. Ad agencies, the drug companies, and the TV networks had lobbied the FDA & Congress for some more rules changes. In August, 1997, they got an early Christmas present.

1992's Prescription Drug User Fee Act was joined by an FDA "clarification" of its 30-year-old drug company advertising regulations. The change loosened up on broadcast advertising. Now, drug companies could advertise on TV without full disclosure of risks & side effects. So long as the commercial mentioned the "major" risks of the drug, along with other sources for information, that was good enough.

Result? Ads for Viagra™ & Claritin™ began running between Burger King™ commercials. The "chosen" drugs (those on TV) began racking up record sales.

"By 1999, the average American was exposed to nine prescription drug advertisements on television every day. The number of television ads increased 40-fold between 1994 and 2000." [1]

Suddenly, anything under the sun was fodder for prime time commercials. Erectile dysfunction, toenail fungus, you name it.

At least they had a sense of humor. Some years later, a new commercial debuted, fretting that their new space age erectile dysfunction product might cause men to experience erections of 4 hours or longer! And THAT, as we all well know, is downright dangerous. "So if that happens to you, call your doctor immediately!"

Footnote:
1 - Abrahamson, p 152

6 - Lucille's Story

Two of my closest friends are Michael & Linda Dlouhy, from Brooksville, Florida.

Linda's grandmother died 20 years ago. Her grandfather was alone in Maine, and, not getting any younger. Over the years, he began to have some health problems. His last 8 years, grampaw spent in Florida, living with Linda's mother as his primary caregiver. He had 9 children, and Lucille was the only one who loved him enough to care for him.

True to the saying, no good deed goes unpunished. Grampaw was always mean to Lucille. I've heard it's pretty normal for the primary caregiver to be treated like crap. And that is how Grampaw treated Lucille.

For instance ... grampaw was incontinent. Lucille told him he needed to wear Depends, so he wouldn't soil the bed every night. But when she put some in his bedroom, he just pulled all the cotton wadding & packing out of them and piled the pieces up on the bed, just to be mean. And he was hell on wheels verbally, too.

Lucille was about 60 at the time. She was a slim, good-looking woman, in excellent health. In her entire life, she had never taken any prescription drugs. But she was under a lot of stress, especially her last 2 years with Gramps. He finally passed away at home in 1996, in Lucille's arms.

Lucille was exhausted, due to the emotional roller-coaster. Immediately after Grampaw's funeral, she went to bed and stayed there for awhile. She felt so bad, she finally went to the doctor. Her blood pressure was up. Big surprise! So the doctor put her on a prescription drug.

And once she got on that drug, Lucille started gaining weight. She gained a LOT of weight. In the next 12 months, she gained 100 pounds. Concerned, of course, she went back to the doctor. And now, she's got a thyroid problem. That required another prescription.

And THAT drug actually stopped her from breathing. Linda went online and found that inability to breathe was one of the "rare side effects." And the antidote was to drink a couple glasses of milk. So Linda gave Lucille some milk, and that dissipated the drug.

Lucille wasn't getting better. In fact, she got worse. Each time she went back to the doctor, she came home with a new prescription. After about 5 years, she was on a total of 15 prescription drugs. And then she had a stroke. It all started with one blood pressure prescription.

This is truly a classic. Lucille had never in her life taken a prescription drug, never been overweight. She started taking 1 drug, which caused some nutrient deficiencies. So her body craved more nutrition. Result? She ate and ate and ate. As she started taking more and more drugs, she got fatter and sicker.

Michael & Linda finally got Lucille to realize that she is responsible for her own health. She stopped going to the doctor for everything. She started taking an excellent multi-nutrient supplement.

Now Lucille is back down to 4 prescription drugs, and she's lost about half the weight-gain. She's on her way to being healthy again. Most people, however, never understand the effect their prescription drugs are having on them.

15

7 – It's Déjà vu All Over Again

What do the following people have in common?

Entertainment:
Jack Webb, Dana Andrews, Fred Astaire, Mary Astor, Ethel Barrymore, George Brent, Claudette Colbert, Gary Cooper, Broderick Crawford, Dan Dailey, Yvonne DeCarlo, Kirk Douglas, Joan Fontaine, Glenn Ford, Arthur Godfrey, Betty Grable, Rita Hayworth, Bob Hope, Alan Ladd, Dorothy Lamour, Fred MacMurray, Barbara Stanwyck, Virginia Mayo, Maureen O'Hara, Gregory Peck, Tyrone Power, Basil Rathbone, Dale Robertson, Rosalind Russell, Ed Sullivan, Robert Taylor, Richard Widmark, Jane Wyman, William Bendix, Perry Como, Bing Crosby, Peggy Lee, Frank Sinatra, Jack Benny, Ray Bolger, George M. Cohan, Claudette Colbert, Gary Cooper, Steve McQueen, Marlene Dietrich, Douglas Fairbanks, Leslie Howard, Hedy Lamarr, Robert Montgomery, Walter Winchell, Amelia Earhart, Eddie Cantor, Groucho Marx, Henry Fonda, Mario Lanza, Jackie Cooper, Dick Van Dyke, & others

Sports:
Joe DiMaggio, Stan Musial, Ted Williams, Mel Ott, Leo Durocher, Frank Gifford, Arnold Palmer, Bob Cousy, Roger Maris, Whitey Ford, Yogi Berra, Mickey Mantle, Bob Lemon, Early Wynn, Red Barber, Dizzy Dean, Lou Gehrig, & others

Politics:
Coolidges, Trumans, Rockefellers, Roosevelts, Vanderbilts, & others

Every one of them – and many more – was featured in cigarettes ads. They appeared in magazines, on ra-

16

dio and TV for Camel™, Chesterfield™, Old Gold™, Lucky Strik™, and numerous other brands. They gushed about how much they loved their cigarette, how smooth and healthful it was.

A 1933 magazine ad noted 21 out of 23 players on the champion New York Giants smoked Camels™ because "It Takes Healthy Nerves To Win the World Series."

"New king-sized Viceroy™ gives you double-barrelled health protection." *Time* magazine, Nov. 9, 1951.

An R J Reynolds ad from 1946:

"Throat Specialist report on 30-Day Test of Camel Smokers — Not one single case of throat irritation due to smoking Camels! Yes, these were findings in a total of 2,470 weekly examinations of hundreds of men and women from coast to coast who smoked only Camels for 30 consecutive days! And the smokers in this test averaged one to two packs of Camels a day! According to a Nationwide Survey: More Doctors Smoke Camels than any other cigarette!"

Many cigarette ads featured middle-aged male doctors, complete with labcoat & stethoscope, healthfully smoking their heads off. Cigarette ads in the 1950s claimed cigarettes help your disposition, improve digestion, provide a lift, ease tension, calm nerves, and keep women thin. In World War II, cigarettes were part in GIs C-rations, to addict GIs and create brand loyalty. By the end of the war, cigarette sales hit an all-time high.

What's The Point?

In the 1920s, 30s, 40s, 50s, & 60s, cigarette ads showed smokers as successful, glamorous, sexy, fun-loving, and athletic … just like the drug ads of today. Celebrities were paid to do commercials … just as the drug companies do today. Doctors were paid to endorse smoking … just as today they are paid to endorse pharmaceuticals. Tobacco companies paid for – and then promoted – scientific research proving that smoking was not a health risk.

You couldn't trust the celebrities, the doctors, the manufacturers, the media, the scientists, or the government regulators back then. What makes you think you can trust them now?

8 - How Your Body Really Works

Imagine your body is a spinning "top", run by a nutrient battery. Your "top" needs a constant flow of the right nutrition to strengthen its immune system, giving it the tools to operate to its potential. When your nutrient battery delivers the right amount of the right juice, then your "top" spins perfectly. You are healthy as a horse.

What if you let the battery charge run down? So your energy lowers. Your functions get erratic. Instead of spinning tightly, you wobble all over. Result? You don't feel so hot.

Running right, your body is a buzz of communication. Microscopic pathways from head to toe hum with metabolic activity. But as your energy level goes down, the strength of action in your metabolic pathways decreases, and your body's communication between organs disappears.

Bad things happen. You get sick. People get dead before their time. To avoid this, you need to restore your natural metabolic pathways. With no toxic interference, given the right nutrients, your body gets rid of the bad stuff. You can get back to the perfect structure you were designed to be.

Proper nutrition brings body normalcy. **It does not target symptoms.** But a raft of symptoms can disappear.

Your ONLY Accurate Gauge of Health

Pain & discomfort are symptoms. They warn you of a problem. They are not illnesses in themselves. To forever get rid of the pain, you must find and cure the cause.

Your body is designed to operate within certain limits. For example, <u>structural limits</u>. No matter how hard you flap your arms, you won't fly. That's a structural limit. And there are <u>functional limits</u>. Drink a few shots of whisky. Chances are, you'll find your functional limits.

But take care of your body, don't push your structural limits, keep that battery juiced up so you function okay, and you'll operate in the normal range. That's called *homeostasis*. The dictionary definition is "the tendency toward a relatively stable equilibrium between interdependent elements."

You want that. It's the ONLY accurate gauge of health. Outside these limits, a million things can go wrong. Symptoms like pain and discomfort say you're *way beyond your limits*. A symptom is information.

Prescription drugs only make things worse. They mask symptoms, so you continue harming yourself. When your foundation is crumbling, you can't just slap on some drugs to cover the cracks. If you live long enough, just the weight of the toxic stuff you're patched up with will kill you.

In football, they call it "misdirection." You send everybody left. The defense follows. But the guy with the ball runs right. And that's where science is. Medical people won't change, because the peer group would laugh at them. Their grants would get cut off. Prescription drug sales would crash. So don't expect help from the academics or the doctors or the drug companies. It won't happen.

It's so obvious…but why don't they get it? (The answer to that question - **$$** - will soon become apparent.) Look at your body. It's not a foot here, a finger there, a heart over there, and a spleen at the other place. They are all connected. Your body is an integrated system.

Remember that definition of *homeostasis*? "The tendency toward a relatively stable equilibrium between *interdependent elements*." That is your body. It is an integrated system. To treat any unwanted condition, you MUST address the whole system.

Unintended Consequences of Statin Drugs

When you take a prescription statin drug to lower cholesterol, it goes ZOOM to your liver and blocks the metabolic pathways there in order to slow cholesterol production. That's precisely how the scientists designed it to work.

But guess what? *Those same metabolic pathways deliver nutrients to your liver.* **They also help direct the toxins away from your liver. And your statin drug puts a stop to ALL of that, not just the cholesterol factory.**

So your cholesterol reading really comes down. But over time, your spinning top slows down, starts to feel REAL wobbly ... and you don't have a clue why that's happening.

Prescription Drugs Don't Cure ANY Disease

They just mask symptoms, so you feel better. Which is not really what you want. The problem hasn't gone away, and it hasn't been addressed. Untreated, it may well escalate in your body and become life threatening.

If you take prescription drugs, you need to get off them over a period of time, to save your health. And repair the damage they've caused. Bottom line, anything you eat or drink must either:

1. Be used to build your body (NUTRIENTS), or

2. Be eliminated through the stomach, the bladder, the lungs and the skin (TOXINS), or

3. Be stored in your body, mainly in the adipose fat and in organs, lymph nodes, glands and joints (TOXINS). These deposits can eventually cause you a world of trouble. Over time, they may threaten your life.

Your body has great capacity to heal, given the proper nutrients. It has very limited ability to deal with a steady stream of contaminants … including prescription or over-the-counter drugs.

Cause And Effect Are Misunderstood

When someone says organisms cause disease, they're flip-flopping cause & effect. When your body is functioning normally, your system won't support malevolent organisms.

Example: there are products to kill parasites in your body. Yes, most of us have them. I live in Florida. We have BUGS! Spray them and kill them, they go away. But since I can't change the environment, they come back.

Likewise, new internal parasite "solutions" don't do a thing. You effectively spray the roaches. And in the process, you toxify your body big-time.

So you get a bunch of long, dead worms in your stool. But in two short weeks, they're back. The reason you have parasites is, you're not in homeostasis. In other words, your body is not in normal function. It's not designed to house parasites. Your body pH is wrong. When you're homeostatic, your parasites won't live. They're gone.

Chemical approaches just don't work. Every symptom comes from one cause: being out of

**homeostasis. If you don't address the problem
nutritionally, you don't address the problem.**

With ANY chemical solution to an invasion, your
body is a battlefield. Good guys fight bad guys. At the end,
what's left? Casualties. Destruction. Good guys die. Bad guys
die. There's no winner.

The medical doctors hope their drugs will kill enough
bad guys so the good guys will win. But they never think
about the mess on the battlefield. Dead bodies everywhere.
And what is a critter's dead body inside your body?

It's a toxin. And those toxins interfere with necessary
nutrient delivery via your metabolic pathways. Result? Sickness. Or worse. So the solution is not chemical. The answer
is absolutely NOT prescription or over-the-counter drugs.

**Your body needs the right nutritional information
to operate optimally.**

I'm not saying that prescription drugs are never called
for. There are rare times when you are in dire straits and you
need some prescription drug to stop a huge threat to your
body. But at the same time, you MUST realize that, over the
long run, you are also causing more harm through nutrient
depletion. Because that is what prescription drugs do.

So your best plan is, increase your nutrient intake
anytime you must take a prescription or over-the-counter
drug. And then get off that drug as soon as possible.

9 - Why Your Body Has Problems

A drug is like the wrong-sized piece in the jigsaw puzzle: it can be forced into place, but you won't have the right picture. That's the problem with drugs. What your body is expecting is raw materials it can use to build. What it gets, in a prescription drug, is a foreign object whose purpose is to STOP the building. So the puzzle picture doesn't look like anything your body is expecting to see.

Good nutrition carries the information your body is starving for. Your body interprets the information and applies it to the various areas that need it. Such products don't coerce or manipulate – they don't force action or reaction. They just offer your body the information it needs to decide how, where, and when to return to normal function.

Drugs, on the other hand, exist ONLY to force action. They take over your normal body function.

Your Metabolic Pathways Are The Key

They deliver information throughout your body. If that information is altered in any way through the use of other substances, or combining substances, this changes and alters the information so it no longer has the intended usefulness to your body.

The moment you combine two substances, you create the characteristics of a third.

For example: hydrogen and oxygen. Both are gases. Combined correctly, they form water. *Water doesn't have the characteristics of oxygen, nor does it have the characteristics of hydrogen.* Yet these two elements make water.

24

Question: When you send chemicals (prescription or over-the-counter drugs) down the same metabolic pathways where your nutrients flow, do you think for one moment that you get the characteristics of *nutrients* at the end?

Answer: No. You don't. But that's where we stop thinking. We just accept that somehow, in this mysterious universe, these principles don't apply to prescription medications. We think they're exempt. We think the doctors know better.

They don't. Doctors are taught how to deal with sickness. They are NOT taught how to create or maintain health. There is a big difference.

Drug nutrient depletion is a huge issue. And it's just added on top of all the other stress factors on your body. Like pollution. And a sedentary lifestyle. As it is, nutrients have largely been strip-mined from our farm soils, so your food is pretty empty. You eat *nutrient-free* fast food at Burger King™, McDonald's™, Pizza Hut™, Taco Bell™. Yummy!

Over Time, Your Body Starts To Break Down

So you take prescription drugs to deal with the results – the diabetes, the high blood pressure, the cholesterol. Or use over-the-counter drugs for your headache or backache.

You're trying to use *pharmaceuticals* to cure *nutritional* deficiencies, in other words. Result? You end up using more energy to get from point A to point B. Your engine is not running efficiently. So just to get the same result you got a few years ago, you have to burn a lot more fuel. You burn a lot more nutrients by using the wrong-sized puzzle piece.

So where in heck are you getting all those extra nutrients?

10 - How Did We Get In This Mess?

Medicine looks at disease like there's something wrong with nature. But it's not nature. It's what we do to it.

Do you know how they make white flour? You start with a wheat grain that has fiber, healthy oils, protein, vitamins & minerals. Then you mill off all that stuff. That leaves you the endosperm with lots of calories, and no nutrition. Grind up the endosperm & bleach it, and you have white flour. It's a nutritional disaster.

But it makes a great insecticide. No kidding. Go out in your yard and catch some bugs and put them in a container with white flour. Put in a little plate of water, so they don't dehydrate. In 24 hours, they'll all be dead.

Anyone for pancakes?

Our nutrient-depleted lifestyle causes diseases like obesity and diabetes, because all the disease-fighting nutrition has been stripped away from our foods.

There's more. Cattle and hens are fed hormones and antibiotics so they grow faster & produce more milk, more meat. We place a much higher value on "convenient" eating as opposed to "healthful" eating.

Insecticides, herbicides, fungicides. Car exhaust, industrial pollution. Heavy metals like mercury, lead, copper, cadimum, aluminum. Dyes, preservatives, drying agents, extenders, binders, fillers. Polish, glue, paint. Hairspray, perfume. Petroleum products, fabric softener, stain remover.

These factors affect all of us. That's why it's not uncommon for something in your body to go wrong. So you go to the doctor. And you get a prescription. But prescription drugs put ALL these other toxins to shame!

Doctors Think Only Some High-Tech, Expensive Equipment Can Diagnose & Treat

Not true.

If that's what you think, and if you believe germs cause disease, then how do you explain our survival until now? Bacteria & viruses are old and tough. They should've killed us off long ago.

A hundred years ago, there weren't any antibiotics. Hardly any prescriptions. Germs were everywhere. Just like they are today. But reality is, you don't just get a bug and die. A baby wouldn't live a week.

The war against disease is continuous in your body. You only know about it if your immune system is weak, and you get symptoms. And when you get symptoms, doctors batch them and give them a name. Drug companies come up with high profit medications to get rid of the symptoms.

Side effects? Oh, well …

"Didn't you read the jar? Didn't you watch the TV commercials? We TOLD you you might get headache, nausea, bloating, loss of vision, sexual side effects, but you have a low risk of experiencing a fatal event."

11 - The Minor Role Of Medicine In Your Health

Most people are born healthy. If not tampered with, they stay healthy throughout life. You seldom need intervention with illnesses, because your body, as well as your mind, can defend and heal itself against most disease and injury.

So medical intervention is the <u>least</u> important of the four factors that determine the state of your health. In 1980, the Centers for Disease Control published data on the top influences on healthfulness in the United States:

1. Lifestyle (51%)
2. Environment (20%)
3. Biologic inheritance (19%)
4. Medical intervention (10%)[1]

Professor Thomas McKeown of Birmingham University says medicine played a very small role in extending Britain's average lifespan the past few centuries. The major factors were improvements in nutrition and public sanitation.[2]

Researchers John & Sonja McKinlay have shown that medical intervention only accounted for 1% to 3.5 % of the increase in the average U.S. lifespan since 1900.[3]

So health depends on prevention, thorough hygiene and good nutrition. When therapy is used, it must deal with the whole person. Treat actual causes – don't just isolate & suppress symptoms. As for prescription & over-the-counter drugs, the "cure" is often worse than the disease.

Result? Collapse. Degenerative disease. And the doctor says, "Gee, did my best. Got him with chemo, radiation, angioplasty, and a heart transplant. Sorry. Must be genetic."

Since They Never Understood The Problem, He's Dead As a Doornail!

If YOU understand, the problem is loss of homeostasis. Hiding symptoms doesn't move you to health. Adding more toxins to your system in the form of prescription or over-the-counter drugs just makes it worse. You can spend a bundle. Get shots, radiation, take pills, torture yourself, sing silly songs, bury a one-eyed toad under a chestnut tree. But until you move back to homeostasis, you're sick – and likely to get worse.

In 1971, President Nixon declared war on cancer in his State of the Union address. Since then, the National Cancer Institute has thrown countless billions into a "medical Vietnam." Over 1,500 Americans will die of cancer today. And tomorrow, next day, every day this year. That's over 550,000 deaths this year. That's 63% more deaths than in 1971, when the War on Cancer began. What happened?

In 1988, the infertility rate for the entire U.S. population was 13.7%. So as many as 1 in 7 of American couples can't reproduce.[4] The Western male's sperm count dropped nearly 50% between 1938 and 1991.[5] That kind of drop in wildlife, we'd expect the species to go extinct.

Not us. We don't see it coming. We just INCREASE toxin intake to make symptoms go away. We crawl along, like the armadillo in the highway, with an 18-wheeler heading right for us. We don't change a thing. And there's no reason on earth to expect that 18-wheeler to change its path.

Footnotes:
1 – "Ten Leading Causes of Death"
2 – McKeown, p 22
3 – McKinlay, p 22
4 - Wood,
5 - Carlsen

12 - You May As Well Use Cocaine!

There used to be a TV commercial with the guy jogging, bragging he just had knee surgery and took a famous name-brand painkiller. Now he can jog miles! He can't feel pain, so it must be OK.

If people believe that garbage, they can hurt themselves. They can cause a lot of damage. You and I know that the painkiller didn't make his knee stronger. It takes time to recover from surgery.

Drugs can make you feel great, because in your body, _they block your metabolic pathways_. They stop the communication between various parts of your body. That's why the pain stops. But the drugs themselves are not a tool your body can use, so they get stored in muscle, tissue, heart, brain.

They stop your body from recognizing symptoms. The problem is still there … nothing has happened to improve your health. But your helpful, legal prescription severs your body's consciousness of pain – just like morphine, valium, or cocaine. Same result.

Biochemical Chaos

Remember: that prescription you're taking is not a "smart bomb." It has a systemic effect, changing cell functions right and left. Changing a single cell function affects your whole body. One prescription drug results in thousands of unwanted biochemical changes. In some cases, you'll immediately notice your new physical problems.

So you see the doctor, and he prescribes Drug #2. So now you multiply. You get tens of thousands of unwanted biochemical changes. And more problems. Back to the doctor. Multiply your new conditions by Drug #3, and you may well wind up with hundreds of thousands of unwanted biochemical changes in your body.

You may not see or feel them immediately. But that doesn't mean they aren't happening.

The average elderly patient is on at least 6 drugs. Look at our elderly population. Is it any wonder so many of them spend 10 or 15 or 20 years suffering all manner of debilitating physical conditions ... and then they die? You've seen it happen, maybe in your own family. Is that the kind of future you want for yourself & your loved ones?

You've probably read of medical journals warning doctors to cut down on prescribing antibiotics, because excessive use has bred "superbugs" that no antibiotic can kill. Not just that. Antibiotics aren't a "smart bomb", either. They kill the good guys, the bacteria necessary for proper digestion, the bacteria that eat up toxins in your system.

The onslaught of chemicals has brought us a catastrophically expensive and ineffective "healing" system, killing and injuring hundreds of thousands of people every year. And still, the costs go up and up and up.

You need a real solution.

Does Your Doctor Have The Answer?

Back to that crucial principle that seems to have been lost on the medical profession: If you don't understand the problem, you can't solve it.

Chances are, you'll make it worse.

"It is simply not possible to identify all the adverse effects of drugs before they are marketed," say three physicians writing in the *New England Journal of Medicine*.[1] In fact, "Overall, 51% of approved drugs have serious side effects not detected prior to approval."[2]

Doesn't that statement astonish you? The implications are incredible.

And yet, despite widespread knowledge in the medical community that half of all new drugs will cause serious side effects, neither the government nor the drug companies systematically collect information on adverse reactions to new drugs. "Even when it is recognized that a new drug will be given to many patients for many years, rarely are systematic post-marketing studies carried out."[3]

If you don't see that anything you eat has a systemic effect, then you can't understand what drugs do. And you can't understand health – how to establish it or how to support it.

Every cell in your body has inherited characteristics which create your structure and control your function. All this information is in your DNA, including optimal levels & ranges of each body function. But there's a catch. If you don't ingest the right materials ... give your body the right *tools* ... your structure won't work right. And drugs won't help you.

Drugs are geared to symptoms. That won't help. You get side effects. You're further from normal function. *ANY product not under your body's control is a drug.* By definition, that's dangerous.

A properly-formulated nutritional product is a tool your body uses to get the right quantity and quality of nutrients. When your body suddenly gets what it's been missing, you can kiss a lot of symptoms good-bye.

Remember – if you don't understand the problem, you can't solve it. We often assume the guy with a ton of facts knows the answers. But as Sherlock Holmes said, "Facts are always convincing. The problem is, we often draw wrong conclusions from facts."

So how did you and I get on our wrong path?

Science is not an altruistic profession. The truth is, scientists are belief-promoters. Their focus? "Name the problem & patent a medicine to stop the symptoms."

The pharmaceutical industry originally took control of hospitals, universities, research and other institutions in the early 1900s. This is documented by medical historian and author, Hans Ruesch, in his book: **Naked Empress or The Great Medical Fraud** (1992). Ruesch documents corruption and fraud in medicine, science, industries, governments, media, and various organizations. Pretty interesting.

Example: "A compilation of the magazine *Advertising Age* showed that as far back as 1948 the larger companies spent for newspapers, radio & magazine advertising the sum total of $1.1 Billion, when the dollar was still worth a dollar. Of this staggering sum the (pharmaceutical) interests controlled about 80%, and utilized it to manipulate public information on health and drug matters - then as now."[4]

The point is, when you understand the politics and money involved, you can make your own decisions based on what you think is best for yourself and your family's health.

How To Know If A Product Is Good

Most people have no idea whether a product they ingest is good for them or not. The decision to take it is based on limited information. Good rule of thumb: If it's food, it has a chance to be good. If it's a drug, what does it really do?

An excellent, first-rate nutritional product must be contaminant-free. It is grown without artificial fertilizers or pesticides. Neither chemicals nor heat are used in the extraction process. It is handled in sterile environments with appropriate containers that don't leach anything into the raw material.

How does this information apply to your drugs? When your body's "nutrient battery" is running right, you have a solid structure. A healthy, enduring structure, based on your body's original blueprint.

The architect didn't design faults. They pop up later. When you ingest stuff that won't sustain health, your structure goes bad. Maybe you'll survive MS or diabetes ... but you sure won't fire on all cylinders.

In fact, your structure alters itself to fit the degenerative mood created by unwanted chemicals.

I've known people who were total non-risk takers. And they think taking prescription drugs is playing it safe. Who do you see who takes a bunch of prescription drugs and then gets well, never needs those drugs again?

The TV commercials say "there's a low risk of side effects." Listen. There is 100% risk that prescription drugs deplete crucial nutrients in your body. Their entire purpose is to STOP your body metabolism from working the way it normally does. And that affects a whole lot more than just the single marker your drug is targeted for.

Many prescription drugs start a nutrient deficiency cycle that can damage your heart. You may even set yourself up for osteoporosis or cancer. Most doctors don't know, because drug companies don't tell them. You need to protect yourself. Learn how these deficiencies occur, and correct them.

Footnotes:
1 – Wood
2 – Moore
3 – Wood
4 - Ruesch

13 - Drugs Can't Fool Your Body

If your car has 14" wheels, it won't take 16" tires. That doesn't mean 16" tires aren't tires. They just aren't designed for your car. It's the same with anything you eat. Your body is expecting nutrients. Drugs are not nutrients. Your body sees the package and realizes it's not a nutrient.

If your body can't recognize it as a nutrient, then it's a poison – not a miracle drug.

If you don't know or value what nutrition is, how can you make drugs that won't poison people? If you don't understand the problem, you can't solve it. *Drugs – ALL drugs – actually mess up your body's metabolic pathways.*

Drugs are toxic. Your body recognizes that. You can't use them. They're stored in muscle and tissue as a toxin. Worse … many drugs are astringent. So they draw fluids from tissue. That brings the swelling down, sure. Tumors may seem to shrink. Cancers might seem to disappear.

Why? Because the fluids are pulled out. And if that was the end of it, great. But it's not. Astringent drugs suck out fluid all over your body. So your liver gets sucked dry. Your organs get dehydrated. And who knows how many toxins you end up with, embedded in your cells, because there's no fluid to transport them out?

Your Problem is Local – But the Effect of Your Drugs Is Systemic

Drugs don't differentiate between the good guys and the bad guys. They don't stop and think. They just suck life out of whatever gets in their way.

If you take any strong astringent over time, you risk pneumonia. Why? Because when you lose liquid from your lung tissue, you get weakness in the cell walls. That opens you up for serious problems, like pneumonia.

Your lymphatic system is a toxic highway, the major transportation system carrying poisons out of your body. If there's no fluid, you get no constant flow of toxins from your body. They stay. That's what you get with ANY drug. It's a compound your body can't recognize, so it gets treated like poison. You're not getting what you think.

You eat. If the body labels it "nutrition," it gets used. But when your body doesn't recognize the stuff, it thinks, "Uh-oh! Poison!" If the garbage can't be moved out of your body, it gets dumped somewhere in your muscle & tissue.

When you take a drug, your body labels it, "Poison." You get miracles because the stuff clogs up your body's metabolic pathways, which blocks you from feeling pain. So you get the illusion, it's helping.

But when your body can't use the stuff, it just gets stored. You will pay, eventually. Some people say, "My doctor wouldn't give me this if it wasn't OK." This is where you must STOP!! Think this through. When you put laboratory chemicals (prescription drugs) into your body, do you think for a moment that your natural immune system just lets all these foreign chemicals pass right on through?

Your body deals with inappropriate information either by precipitating it or removing it from your system. When you feed your body a daily dose of laboratory chemicals, you overburden your system. In time, the excess precipitates to various organs, gumming up the works.

Your body degenerates when it loses its ability to communicate via the immune system. Which leads to arthritis, kidney stones, gallstones, heart attack, etc. Drugs do a great job of severing communication between the body and consciousness. So you get this feel-good result – until they start precipitating out in various organs. Then you get degenerative disease, maybe early death.

Some Amazing Numbers

According to the *Journal of the American Medical Association* (JAMA) of April 14, 1998, "Adverse drug reactions are the fourth leading cause of death in America. Reactions to prescription and over-the-counter medications kill far more people annually than all illegal drug use combined."

Researchers estimated that 106,000 Americans a year die from appropriately administered, FDA-approved prescription drugs. That's more deaths than the annual total for AIDS, suicide, & homicide combined. It's 290 body bags a day. Another 40,000 a year die from over-the-counter drugs.

A report by the General Accounting Office showed that 51.5% of all drugs introduced between 1976 and 1985 had to be re-labelled because of serious adverse reactions found after their sale. Reactions included heart, liver and kidney failure, foetal toxicity and birth defects, severe blood disorders, respiratory arrest, seizures and blindness. The changes to the labelling either restricted a drug's use or added major warnings. [1]

It gets worse. Many drug reactions go unnoticed. In *Controversies in Therapeutics* (1980), Dr Leighton Cluff comments: "National Health statistics do not reflect the magnitude of the problem of drug-induced diseases. A death certificate may indicate that a person died of renal failure, but it may not state that the disease was caused by a drug."[2]

As you can imagine, there are a lot of problems in distinguishing toxic reactions from underlying diseases. Many toxic reactions mirror common illnesses. Others have a silent nature. If not specifically looked for, they may not be found (e.g., kidney and liver damage). And, of course, many consumers are on multi-drug regimes, making it tough to figure which toxin caused the suspected reaction.

Most adverse reactions to drugs go unreported, so the official estimates are only the tip of the iceberg.

Yet, many people never realize they have a problem. Why? Because drug toxicity interferes with perception. So a person on drugs often doesn't know how sick she is. Result? Our systems get overwhelmed. With some illnesses, doctors now say toxins alter the DNA. That's what they call, "spontaneous mutation." But remember how those toxins got into your body in the first place?

How Prescription Drugs Stop Your Body's Critical Actions

You and every other living organism have metabolic pathways that must be executed as intended. All your organs, from your brain down to the simplest cell, communicate with each other via these biochemical pathways.

A drug's chemical make-up messes up your body's metabolic pathways. That's what a toxin DOES.

Prescription drugs are designed to alter or stop accurate communication between organs. That's how they control your blood-sugar level, for instance. So when you take prescription drugs, your body won't work right. That's the definition of a toxin.

Your body gets data from its environment, from bread, water, sunshine, whatever. This is the foundation. If the data is pure, your body absorbs and uses it 100%. No need to store excess junk in the garbage pits (your cells).

Your body is like the building. A facade. Its foundation is built on nutrients. Your body takes information from what you feed it. Eat beef from a cow shot up with hormones, and your body takes both the nutrients & the chemicals. It'll use what it can.

The rest gets poured in a toxic dump somewhere in your cells!

Why? Whatever you eat, your body requires a certain presentation. Otherwise, your body doesn't know what it is. So when you eat something your body doesn't recognize, it gets stored. And those poisons build and build.

So prescription drugs deplete the very nutrients your body needs to repair the organ or system the drug is supposed to "cure". For instance, statin drugs lower your CoQ10 level. CoQ10 is a critical nutrient to repair your heart and to bring energy to your body. Lacking CoQ10, you'll often feel like you're "running on empty".

In time, good nutrition helps the body handle problems. Prescription drugs suppress symptoms and damage your system. The scientists shoot at what they can see – that single marker. But that's a symptom. The true source of the problem is deeper. Drugs just plaster the walls while the foundation crumbles.

Footnotes:
1 – "FDA Drug Review Post-Approval Risks 1976-85", p 33
2 – Cluff, p 44

14 - More Evidence Against Prescription Drugs

If prescription drugs are so good, where are all the healthy drug takers?

The only ones I see are on the TV commercials. Drug companies claim their products lower your cholesterol, regulate your blood-sugar, make your heart work better, end clinical depression, reverse osteoporosis, eliminate allergies, calm your children, etc., etc., etc.

Wonderful! So where are all the healthy medicated customers in REAL life?

If drugs are good for you, there should be hundreds of thousands of happy, healthy, athletic drug takers right now. They'd be mentally sharp, with low body fat, high bone density, healthy digestive tracts, healthy blood chemistry, vibrant skin, high energy, excellent moods, etc. Where are they?

More and more, the advertising & personal message from drug companies and doctors is becoming clear: to be healthy, you need to get on their products and STAY on them for the rest of your life. But who do you know who's taking 12 prescriptions and has a clean bill of health? A common observation is, the more prescriptions a person takes, the longer they take them, the worse their health. Do you see a lot of exceptions to this rule?

Here are some of the symptoms you may have noticed in people taking multiple prescriptions:

- overweight

- chronically fatigued
- depressed
- sickly in appearance
- mentally clouded
- multiple blood chemistry problems
- weak immune system
- low bone density
- emotionally unstable.

Stop by a local health club. Ask some folks what prescription drugs they take to be so healthy. THAT should get you an interesting response!

The U.S. accounts for 50% of the total world spending on drugs. And yet the World Health Organization ranks the U.S. as the 37[th?] most healthy country. [1] How can that be, if prescription drugs are such a health boon?

Why Does The FDA Approve Drugs?

Call me cynical, but I think a big reason the FDA approves any drug is that by the 1992 Prescription Drug User Fee Act of Congress, drug companies now PAY the FDA for this service. And the FDA absolutely does NOT get paid to find problems with any drugs. If YOU got paid for one thing and NOT paid for the other thing, which one would YOU do?

Each prescription drug targets one measurable marker, like cholesterol level or bone density. If a drug can positively alter *any* measurable marker - and the number of immediate fatalities is statistically small enough – then the FDA declares it "safe & effective" and the TV commercials crank up. Ka-ching! Another two million dollars a day!

No doubt, the drug moves that marker. **But every drug has a systemic effect, and these systemic effects are not accurately measured (or admitted) in clinical trials.**

Statin drugs lower bad cholesterol levels by limiting the liver's ability to create ALL cholesterol ... including "good" cholesterol & critical hormones your body makes from cholesterol.[2] So you get one measurable, positive effect and your body's health gets trashed a hundred other ways ... like blocking your sex drive, for instance.

If the drug moves the marker, it gets FDA approval. Other effects to your body aren't considered. If a clinical trial results in severe effects on some participants, no one from the FDA sees it. A drug company can simply dismiss those participants and finish the trial. Do we wind up with extremely toxic drugs getting quick approval? Absolutely.

More deaths & injuries are caused each year by prescription drugs than in any U.S. war since World War II.

The April, 1998, article in the *Journal of the American Medical Association* admits 100,000 Americans a year die from properly-administered prescription drugs and 2 million more are injured. Plus another 40,000 or so killed by over-the-counter pain medications.

And that figure is only what they can see! It does not include future fatalities and debilitation due to the nutrient deficiencies caused by every single one of these drugs. For most people, the effects of these nutrient deficiencies take time to become apparent. And rarely will they be traced back to the prescription drug.

But *every* pharmaceutical causes nutrient deficiencies. It's not hard to see the big picture, considering about 2/3 of the U.S. population takes prescription or over-the-counter drugs (pain relief, etc.) or both.

Miracle Drugs? Healthy? Not Hardly.

The obvious counter to this argument is that people only take prescription drugs after they're already sick. Not so:

Statins are now being pushed onto healthy people with cholesterol levels of 115, as a preventative measure. "Dr. Robert A. Rizza, vice president of the American Diabetes Association (ADA), recommends statin drugs to diabetic patients without a shred of proof that they help", just in case some benefits are someday discovered![3]

Now consider this. Donating at least $500,000 each to the American Diabetes Association are: Novartis, Merck, Parke-Davis, Pfizer, SmithKline Beecham, Takeda, Bayer, Aventis & Eli Lilly. [4] All of them are monster pharmaceuticals. Does this explain the ADA's recommendation.

Statins are designed to interfere with normal liver function. That's how they change the cholesterol marker. Side effects, anyone? Recommending someone without a cholesterol problem get on this drug is really not in the best interest of people's health.

The Vicious Cycle Kicks In

And when they get on the statins, and the side effects kick in, they'll go to a medical doctor and get diagnosed with some new disease or condition. For which they'll need to add another prescription drug. In marketing, this is called "upselling the customer" - when the same customer buys more stuff, you increase your profit margin.

So it's one prescription on top of another, until something breaks ... usually the patient. Result? You get financial hardship for many, chemical toxicity & nutrient depletion for all. By the time a typical patient finally dies from complications caused by the prescription drugs, they may have transferred a fortune to the doctors & the chemical companies. Multiply that number if "heroic drugs" are prescribed during the patient's last surviving days, weeks, or months.

Again, the FDA does not monitor drug testing. So how often do you think the drug companies test prescription drugs for dangerous interactions with other drugs? Maybe some do. But there are a lot of drug companies. It's an unnecessary expense in getting the product to market. I'll bet a lot of them *never* do such testing.

So the FDA approves drug A for one thing, and drug B for another. But did anybody ever test what happens when both are taken together? The combination is often toxic. Many prescription drug combinations are fatal. Others just destroy a liver or pancreas or heart, or some other little organ.

So Why Are Prescription Drugs So Popular?

They are very profitable. Once the formula has been settled on, what do you think it costs to mix the chemicals for a bottle of pills? Not much, that's for sure. The raw ingredients often cost next to nothing. A common mark-up can easily be 1,000% or 5,000% or 10,000%. In other words, that $50 prescription bottle you bought at the drugstore can easily have 5¢ or 1¢ or 1/2¢ of raw materials in it!

45

The news media get millions in drug advertising. The doctors get free vacations, "consulting fees," and other bribes to prescribe brand-name drugs. It's profitable for everyone except you. Your health gets worse. Your debt gets worse. Your insurance rates skyrocket.

"Drug interactions remain a problem. Expected toxic effects from marketed drugs, even when used as directed, is estimated to rank among the top 10 causes of death in the US and is estimated to cost more than $30 billion annually."[5]

Is This Logical To You?

Is your body the same as your neighbor's?

In fact, is there anyone else on earth who has the same metabolism as you do, who has eaten the same diet as you have, who has been exposed to the same amounts of the same environmental toxins as you have?

If you go have bloodwork done and the doctor tells you that you have high cholesterol or high blood-sugar or any of several dozen other measurably abnormal readings ... do you think YOUR readings are exactly the same as the other 50 high blood-sugar or high cholesterol cases your doctor treats? You KNOW the answer to that.

So Here's a Real Timesaver for Your Doctor ...

Why do doctors generally practice "standard dosing?" In other words, chances are if your doctor handles 50 high blood-sugar cases, each of those cases gets prescribed the same amount of the same medication.

You KNOW those readings aren't all the same, the body blood-sugar levels aren't all the same. The need isn't all the same. And yet the prescription for each IS the same: same drug, same amount. Does this make sense to you?

And when they "standard dose," of course, that dose must be high enough to treat the worst case. So if you're just a borderline case affected by the problem, you are getting WAY more drug than you need.

Does this sound like the act of a profession that is really concerned with getting you the best result with the least amount of toxic exposure to you? The beauty of "standard dosing" is, no thought is involved. One size fits all. If you have x blood-sugar or $2x$ or $3x$ or $4x$, it is all the same. You get the same amount of prescription medication.

Now ... one of the reasons these meds are by prescription only is their toxicity. You can't buy them over-the-counter because they are dangerous. And yet, many doctors prescribe the same dose for everybody, no matter how mild or how severe their problem is. Draw your own conclusions.

Do Prescription Drugs Have a Place?

Sure. They are for short-term interventions to save a life while you change your diet, nutrition, & lifestyle. That's a reasonable, legitimate use. When you take prescription drugs long-term, you'll be worse than when you started.

But watch the TV commercials. Short-term use is not how these drugs are promoted. Statins & other drugs are pushed as lifetime medications. Diet, nutrition & exercise are avoided. The result is that patients are told drugs are the only answer.

"Death By Medicine" Online Report

A recent study shows a larger picture of the injury and death by medical errors in the U.S. Seven years of research reviewing thousands of studies show that medical errors are the number one cause of death and injury in the U.S. **According to the NIA's report, over 784,000 people die annually due to medical mistakes. Heart disease deaths in 2001 claimed 699,697; cancer deaths claimed 553,251.**[6]

Do Your Own Research

It's easy these days to find just about any information you want. Just go to:

http://www.google.com/

and type in your question. Make it as specific as you can. You'll probably get 100s or 1000s of pages of results. Read the entries linked in the first page or two. If the question you asked reflects exactly what you want to know, then you will learn a lot about what you are interested in.

1 http://www.photius.com/rankings/who_world_health_ranks.html
2 Pomper
3 Mundell, p 39
4 Adams
5 Friedman
6 Null

15 - Drug-Caused Nutrient Deficiencies

Have you noticed memory, hair, or hearing loss? Or fatigue? Muscle weakness? Anemia? Depression? Are prescription drug side effects damaging your heart? Setting you up for osteoporosis, or even cancer?

I know this is very, very hard for you to believe. But here is the truth: ALL prescribed drugs and over-the-counter medications actually *create* disease.

That's *crazy*, you say? You figure I must be some wild-eyed whacko for making a statement like that? The drug companies wouldn't put out a product that knowingly creates disease, would they? And surely, your doctor wouldn't go along with it?

It's critical to your health that you really understand how your body works ... and how a drug works.

Look: Your body's blueprint doesn't say, "When you're 40, your eyesight will go bad. You'll get MS, diabetes, and high blood pressure. At 50, arthritis."

Your Body's Blueprint Is Perfect

NO genetic deformities. Your body's immune system is perfect to stop bad conditions. It has to be, because Mother Nature is one big destruction machine. You wouldn't survive ten seconds without your immune system.

Our immune system only stops working if we block it with poisons and toxins. Which we do. In the past hundred years, we've just about improved ourselves to death. Our food is processed, not raw. We use plastic, not wood. We have poisons in our air, water, food, clothing, furniture, and homes. We now have inescapable daily contact with – and ingestion of – toxins way beyond our understanding.

Listen: your body is amazing. You can handle toxic stuff. Everything you take in is somewhat benign – IF you're operating right. If you get a bit of arsenic, your body can remove it. **But if you ingest toxins every day, as most of us do, you will eventually have some problems.**

So let's say you go to the doctor, because you don't feel so good. And the doctor sends you to have your blood work done. The tests come back. One or more of those numbers – *"markers"*, as they're called by the scientists - is too high, or too low. So your doctor writes you a prescription.

How Your Prescription Drugs Actually Work

The intended purpose of any drug is to get that marker into its proper range … in other words, to get rid of a symptom. No drug cures anything. And as drugs get rid of your symptoms, they also rob your body of vitamins, minerals, & antioxidants. Here's how:

Scientists design a drug to target a single marker in your body, like cholesterol level or insulin level or plaque or stomach acid or bacteria or allergens or tumor growth or … the list goes on and on. So you have a limited, local, measurable problem. And the scientists come up with a chemical concoction to change the marker reading for that problem.

Let's say that through air, water, or food pollution, you ingest more toxins than your body can dispose of. Part of what those toxins do in your body is, they interfere with:

- nutrient absorption and/or
- metabolism and/or
- nutrient storage and/or
- nutrient transport and/or
- nutrient use by cells

The scientists understand that *something* has moved some marker reading in your body away from its appropriate level. So they design a drug to change it back, to reverse the process. The way ANY drug changes a marker in your body is by interfering with:

- nutrient absorption and/or
- metabolism and/or
- nutrient storage and/or
- nutrient transport and/or
- nutrient use by cells

Interesting, isn't it?

And HERE is the problem:

This "wonder" drug does not affect just that single target marker that uses your metabolic pathways for nutrient absorption, storage, transport, etc. Your whole body uses this communication system to receive the nutrients it requires for normal function.

The result is, 100% of the time, your drug "treatment" has a *systemic* effect. Not only do you get the reaction the drug was designed for ... you get lots of other

reactions, and all the immediate side effects they cause ... and all the "nutrient deficiency" side effects that may stay hidden for weeks or months or years.

Did any doctor or pharmacist ever tell you this? Serious symptoms often hide until you have heart disease or cancer. Isn't that a kick in the butt? Most pharmacists & doctors don't know the size of the problem, because pharmaceutical companies don't tell them. So how could patients know that their drugs are depleting their bodies of nutrients?

You need to protect yourself. Depleted nutrient levels lead to lowered immune system function, and a ton of other problems. Learn how these deficiencies occur, and take steps to correct them.

Drug-induced nutrient depletions may be news to you.
.

Ask the drug companies, and they'll tell you nutrient depletion isn't an issue. It's not happening. And THAT answer is BS. Did you really expect drug companies to pay for studies that verify that their drug is causing nutrient depletions?

Health Sciences Institute research (September, 1999) concludes that **medicating one problem can lead to a series of additional problems caused by the nutrient-depleting effects of the initial medication. This generates more prescriptions, which create more nutrient deficiencies. Talk about a vicious cycle!**

Consider antibiotics. They deplete helpful bacteria. Women on antibiotics may develop Candida, including vaginal yeast infections. A doctor may then prescribe more medications to combat the yeast. This cycle can lead to immune system disturbance. Antibiotics also deplete B vitamins, nec-

52

essary for 100s of biological processes, including proper nervous system functioning.

Result? Another array of drug "solutions." It's like *"Alice in Wonderland."*

The elderly often suffer nutritional deficiencies. Taking multiple drugs adds to their problem. Plus, the elderly often use non-prescription drugs like non-steroidal anti-inflammatories or antacids. They don't realize these drugs can make them deficient in calcium, phosphorus, folic acid, iron, magnesium, etc.

How fast do depletions happen? Depends on your lifestyle, diet, stress level, toxic level of your environment, & your nutritional status before the drugs. Everybody is different. There's no set rule.

Again, every single prescription or over-the-counter medication you take does its job by interfering with nutrient absorption, storage, transport, or metabolism. So every single pill you take or medication you drink causes one or multiple nutrient depletions.

That is EVERY drug, including but not limited to:

- anabolic steroids
- antacids
- anti-anxiety agents
- antibiotics
- anticonvulsants
- anti-diabetic drugs
- anti-fungals
- antihistamines
- anti-inflammatory drugs

- anti-Parkinson's Disease drugs
- anti-protozoals
- antiviral drugs
- bronchodilators
- cardiovascular drugs
- chemotherapy drugs
- cholesterol-lowering drugs
- electrolyte replacement: timed release potassium chloride
- female hormones
- gout medications
- laxatives
- psychotherapeutic drugs
- thyroid medications
- ulcer medications
- miscellaneous drugs

Examples of Drug-Caused Nutrient Deficiencies

1. **You take a medication to slow down heart rhythms and improve blood flow.** Two of the nutrients often depleted by these meds are calcium & magnesium, the 2 essential minerals that make your heart beat regularly.

So when you get to the emergency room on some prescription drug, the ER doctors don't understand how you can be going back into an irregular rhythm. Of course, it's because you're depleted of calcium & magnesium.

So what does the doctor do? He gives you MORE drugs. This slows your heart down for awhile. But 2 months later, you're back, heart beating like crazy. NOW what does your doctor do? Increase the medication! Which puts you in a horrible vicious cycle. You wind up with even more complications ... all because the drugs are leeching the nutrients from your system.

2. Aspirin depletes your body of Vitamin C, folic acid, iron, & various amino acids. Many people take aspirin daily, for heart disease. If you're not supplementing, then the "cure" may be worse than the disease.

3. Many over-the-counter & prescription pain relievers, corticosteroids, sulfa drugs, antibiotics, diuretics, oral contraceptives & others cause folic acid deficiency. This B vitamin may be the most common nutrient deficiency in North America. Unless you eat lots of spinach, broccoli, beans, beets, yeast, eggs and meats (like liver & kidneys on a daily basis), you probably need a folic acid supplement.

Only about 25% of the US adults take folic acid supplements. Folic acid lowers homocysteine level, helping prevent heart disease, stroke, birth defects, and maybe osteoporosis & Alzheimer's.

Symptoms of folic acid deficiency:

- elevated homocysteine
- anemia
- headaches
- fatigue
- depression
- hair loss
- insomnia
- increased susceptibility to infection

Folic acid helps relieve arthritic pain, but many common arthritis drugs deplete folic acid. The cells of your intestinal lining have a special need for folic acid because of their

their high rate of replication; yet sulfasalazine, a drug commonly prescribed for colitis, can cause a deficiency of folic acid.

It's likely that 1000s of heart disease & stroke deaths could be prevented with adequate folic acid, at least 400 mcg. Those who need it most include millions of users of anti-inflammatory drugs and oral contraceptives.

4.   Many drugs deplete CoEnzyme Q10. Certain anti-depressants, anti-psychotic drugs, cholesterol-lowering statin drugs, beta-blockers, anti-diabetic drugs, anti-hypertension drugs & others cause a CoEnzyme Q10 deficiency.

Your body manufactures CoQ10 for brain health, energy production and protection against free radical damage. CoQ10 is critical in the synthesis of ATP, our "energy molecule", the chemical fuel used by all cells.

Some studies suggest congestive heart failure & cardiomyopathy are coenzyme Q10 deficiency diseases. But one side effect of these prescription drugs is that they interfere with your body's production of CoQ10. This depletion can be very serious in the elderly, because aging already depletes CoQ10. CoQ10 deficiency may result in Alzheimer's or Parkinson's Disease.

Symptoms of CoQ10 deficiency:

- angina
- cardiac arrhythmias
- mitral valve prolapse
- high blood pressure
- stroke
- gum disease

- low energy – feels like you're "running on empty"
- a weak immune system.

Most doctors have even heard of CoQ10. They don't know that declining CoQ10 levels as we age lead to disease susceptibility. Heart patients, diabetics, and almost everyone approaching retirement age critical needs more CoQ10.

Older persons in good health have difficulty in synthesizing CoQ10, so there is a real danger that the cholesterol lowering drugs, while perhaps reducing the bad cholesterol count, could be damaging the heart's ability to function effectively because of a deficit of CoQ10. How ironic is that?

5. Many commonly prescribed drugs deplete magnesium: oral contraceptives & other estrogens, statin drugs, various antibiotics, diuretics, many heart medications, corticosteroids, & others.

Magnesium deficiency may result in:

- atherosclerosis
- heart attack
- hypertension
- stroke
- life-threatening cardiac spasm (when magnesium levels fall too low, excess calcium enters the heart muscle cells, resulting in a dangerous cramp)
- leg cramps
- insomnia
- restlessness
- irritability
- nervousness
- anxiety
- depression

- fatigue
- osteoporosis
- migraines
- PMS

According to a US Department of Agriculture survey: 75% of Americans consume less than the RDA of magnesium. Magnesium deficiency encourages osteoporosis, cognitive problems & blood sugar regulation. Lack of magnesium can also trigger heart attacks, hypertension and strokes.

Supplementing with magnesium can reduce a host of cardiovascular complications:

- Like aspirin, magnesium inhibits blood clotting
- Like Coumadin™, magnesium thins the blood
- Like Procardia™, a Calcium channel blocker, magnesium prevents excess calcium uptake
- Like Vasotec™, an ACE inhibitor, magnesium relaxes blood vessels

6.   Zinc can also be depleted by a variety of drugs, including carticosteroids, oral contraceptives, oral estrogens, ACE inhibitors, diuretics, cholesterol-lowering drugs, & anti-ulcer drugs. Zinc deficiency is rampant in the United States. It increases with age due to poor absorption and the inadequate diet of many elderly.

Symptoms of a zinc deficiency:

- slow wound healing
- poor sense of smell & taste
- problems with skin, hair and nails (zinc is highly concentrated in skin, hair and nails)
- low immune response and frequent infections

- night blindness
- excessive sensitivity to light
- depression
- lethargy
- anemia
- menstrual & fertility problems
- male sterility
- various pregnancy complications
- joint pain

Zinc deficiency affects the activity of almost all enzymes in the body, as well as the synthesis of various hormones and insulin receptors. White spots on fingernails are a telltale sign of zinc deficiency.

Zinc deficiency causes your arteries to become hard, brittle and often inflamed instead of soft and flexible. When this happens, your body may coat them with calcium and fatty plaques to prevent rupture of the arteries.

The plaque reduces the interior artery diameter, raising blood pressure. More pressure is needed to force blood through the smaller diameter arteries. Deficiencies of copper, zinc, bioflavinoids, vitamins C and E and other nutrients contribute to this problem.

And once again, you wind up in the "vicious prescription cycle."

How Common Blood Pressure Drugs Work

It's estimated that 50 million Americans have high blood pressure. (Many don't know it.) The higher your blood pressure, the greater your risk of stroke, heart attack or heart failure. Lower your blood pressure to reduce the risk. Your doctor usually prescribes a combination of drugs to lower blood pressure, including:

- **Diuretics** - These help your body get rid of salt and water. They cause sodium, potassium, magnesium, & zinc deficiencies

- **Beta-blockers** - These slow down your heart, reducing its workload. They also lower an important hormone, which opens the blood vessels, making it easier for the heart to work. These drugs cause Coenzyme Q10 & melatonin deficiencies.

- **Calcium-Channel Blockers** - These open up the blood vessels making it easier for the heart to work.

- **Angiotensin Converting Enzyme (ACE) inhibitors** - These drugs prevent a hormone being released in your body, helping to open up the blood vessels.

- **Alpha Blockers** - These work by blocking receptors in the blood vessels, lowering blood pressure.

- **Centrally acting drugs** - These work through the brain to lower blood pressure

- **Sympathetic nerve inhibitors** - Sympathetic nerves go from the brain all over the body, including the arteries. They can cause the arteries to constrict, raising blood pressure. These drugs stop the nerves from constricting blood vessels, reducing blood pressure.

- **Blood vessel dilators** - These can cause the muscle in the walls of the blood vessels (especially the arterioles) to relax, allowing the vessel to dilate (widen).

Many doctors will tell you that these treatments must be continued the rest of your life. They don't tell you ... they probably don't even realize ... that each pill you take depletes nutrients from your body.

How These Prescriptions Actually CAUSE High Blood Pressure

Anything not a nutrient is treated by your body as a toxin. Many toxins cannot be eliminated. That's how your prescription drugs can build up and damage the kidneys' ability to regulate your body's water balance, leading to water retention, salt retention and high blood pressure.

Ultimately, people who take drugs like diuretics over time may begin to move into degenerative conditions. Why? Because the drug removes fluid from the tissues. Fact is, you're a bag of fluid. You need that fluid to survive. Less bodily fluid means that MORE toxins will not be removed from your body ... instead, they will be deposited in the soft tissue (brain, heart, other organs).

Drug companies are not required to do nutrient depletion studies, and the funding for such research is difficult to obtain. If you are taking or have taken any prescription or over-the-counter medication regularly, it's important to take nutritional supplements to counteract the nutrient deficiencies caused by the medication.

There are now over 13,000 prescription drugs and hundreds or thousands of over-the-counter drugs. Americans eat over 3 BILLION prescriptions a year! Not a single one of them is a body-building nutrient. Each one of them does its job by STOPPING some normal, automatic body function.

And each one of them actually affects your whole body, stopping many more functions than just the intended one.

Which means that each of these drugs causes one or more nutrient deficiencies somewhere in your body. You need to act to protect your health.

This is by no means a comprehensive discussion of drug-caused nutrient deficiencies. For the most complete record, check *"The Drug-Induced Nutrient Depletion Handbook"* in the "Recommended Vendors" section.

Conclusion? Tto avoid or reverse nutrient depletion, you should take a strong daily dose of a high-quality, full-spectrum, nutrient-dense product. Also, figure what specific supplements you may need, (magnesium, CoQ10, etc.) and add these individually.

16 - Follow The Money Trail

Drug companies make more money than banks, more money than oil companies, more money than Ford or GM. The only mass-market product more profitable than prescription drugs is software. What drugs & software have in common is a dirt-cheap price for the raw material, and an enormous mark-up to the consumer. Mark-ups of 1000%, 5000%, 10,000% and more are pretty standard.

Example: a 1-year dose of Searle's Celebrex^{TM} pain reliever costs $900. A one-year dosage of generic ibuprofen is $24. Raw material cost is about the same. And many people say they get better results with generic ibuprofen.

Deep pockets in the pharmaceutical industry include:

1. powerful drug companies
2. medical technology companies
3. special interest groups with vested interest in the business of medicine

They all fund medical research, support medical schools & hospitals, and advertise in medical journals. With their enormous resources, they can buy as many scientists and academics as they want, who will do studies & write articles. Writing or speaking out against any of the drug company products would certainly be the kiss of death financially for any of these people supported by pharmaceutical dollars.

Nothing Wrong With Making A Profit ...

In 2003, health care spending in the United States reached $1.7 trillion, 4.3 times the amount spent on national defense. In 2003, the United States spent 15.3% of its Gross

Domestic Product (GDP) on health care. It is projected that the percentage will reach 18.7% in 10 years. Between 1995 and 2002, the average increase for drug expenditures was 15% higher than for any other type of health expenditure.[1]

Employment dropped in 2001, the stock market plunged, and Fortune 500 company profits declined by 53%, the 2nd biggest profit dive ever for the Fortune 500. But the top 10 U.S. drug companies increased profits by 33%.[2] That is a profit of 18.5 cents for every $1 of sales, which was 8 times higher than the median for all Fortune 500 industries, easily surpassing the next most profitable industry, which was commercial banking with a 13.5% return on revenue.[3]

In the US, our lifestyle is the envy of the world, because of business. Business has made our country prosperous. We owe a huge debt to our entrepreneurs..

BUT ... people must take responsibility for themselves and their families. Prescription drugs have one of the highest profit margins of any product in any market. Which means there is a LOT of incentive for people in that industry to ignore or even SMASH any kind of negative comment about their products. The question is, are they more concerned about the drug company's future and their own future ... or about your future & your family's future? Are you willing to let THEIR desires decide YOUR future?

How Drug Company Ad Dollars Compare ...

Vioxx™, an arthritis drug sold by Merck & Company, was the most-heavily advertised prescription drug in 2000. Merck spent $160.8 million to promote Vioxx to consumers - more than PepsiCo spent to advertise Pepsi, more than Budweiser spent to advertise beer. Vioxx sales quadrupled $330 million in 1999 to $1.5 billion in 2000.[4]

British pharmaceutical GlaxoSmithKline spent $417 million on consumer advertising in 2000 - more than any other company on earth.[5]

Annually, drug companies spend billions on TV commercials and print media. They spend over $12 billion a year handing out drug samples and employing sales forces to influence doctors to promote specifically branded drugs. The drug industry employs over 1,200 lobbyists, including 40 former members of Congress. Drug companies have spent close to a billion dollars since 1998 on lobbying. In 2004, drug companies and their officials contributed at least $17 million to federal election campaigns.[6]

The Watchdog

The Food & Drug Administration is the government agency charged with approving new drugs and monitoring the safety of all drugs on the market. Some numbers that affect FDA effectiveness:

In 2003, as the drug industry figured out ways to spend its promotional budget of about $12 BILLION, the FDA safety section, which tracks whether drugs are hurting consumers, had a budget of $15 million.[7] That's less than 10% of what Merck spent just to advertise Vioxx[TM] in 2001.

In fact, the entire FDA safety budget is about 1/100th of 1% of the promotional budget of the drug companies!!!

Watchdog? More like a chihuahua in an elephant stampede.

The Source of Patient Group Funding?

Drug companies sponsor "patient groups" that consume whatever drug the company is pushing. Example: the non-profit group CHADD (Children and Adults with Attention Deficit Disorder), which gives info on using Ritalin and other psychotropic meds to control hyperactive kids, is partly funded by Ritalin's manufacturer - Novartis.

The Boots company, which manufactures a thyroid product, has provided 60% funding for the American Thyroid Association.

People go to patient groups for help with some awful condition. Their illusion is that the people in these groups are peers with experience, who will be able to help them make choices. Little do they know the group has been co-opted by a manufacturer to act as an advertising agent. There's no law against this, by the way. It's just another example of why it's so important to control your health to the greatest degree possible, so you don't fall victim to the drug companies.

Self-Prescriptions

Americans will spend over *$500 billion* on drugs this year - not including the extra $100 billion estimated for the Medicare drug benefit program. Spending on prescription drugs is now the fastest growing portion of healthcare spending in the United States.[8]

And a big reason it's growing so fast is that patients see a drug they like in a TV ad, and they go to their doctor for a prescription. More often than not, the doctor will comply. So why would a doctor base prescriptions on requests of patients, who have no medical training? Simple answer: it's easier, less hassle, & less time-consuming to just give people what they want. That is certainly the path of least resistance, which is what most of us take most of the time.

Where Magazines Get Their Profit

Media wants 2 things. #1 is to strongly serve their subscribers' interests and to build a large subscriber base because people love the publication. #2 is to attract big advertisers as a result of #1. In many cases, the actual survival of a publication depends on ad dollars from the drug companies. With so much at stake, can you rely on the truth of what you read or see in the media? Consider:

▸ Millions of dollars of drug ad money go into the American Psychiatric Association 's publications, conferences, continuing education programs, and seminars. 15-20% of APA income comes directly from drug ads in APA journals.[9]

And when those journals write about those drugs, do you imagine the tone is generally positive or negative?

▸ Doctors with conventional Western medical views and against alternative medicine are more likely to publish papers and be on editorial boards of scientific journals than doctors with different philosophies.[10]

Most medical journals get big drug company ad dollars. Do you think they'll ever publish articles or studies recommending alternative medicine over drugs and surgery?

▸ A former editor of the *Journal of the American Medical Association* (JAMA) alleged that Pfizer stopped $250,000 worth of advertising because an article appearing in JAMA had cast one of their drugs in an unfavorable light.[11]

▶ In 1992, *Annals of Internal Medicine* published a study critical of the pharmaceutical industry. Drug ads in the journal declined considerably and stayed low for months.[12]

Many medical journals struggle financially. Do you think they ever kill articles that might annoy an advertiser?

▶ Paid drug ads are the #1 source of income for the *Journal of the American Medical Association.*

▶ 15-20% of the American Psychological Association's (APA) income comes from drug ads in its journals.[13]

But drug advertising doesn't just dominate medical journals. It dominates publications across the board. Take a look at popular consumer publications like *Readers' Digest*, and you'll find many more words in the drug ads than in all the rest of the publication combined.

Put yourself in their shoes. Yes, they want to serve your best interests. But they MUST serve the drug companies' best interests, or they've got money trouble ... maybe out of business. If you rely on any of these publications to be a whistleblower against their advertisers, to protect YOUR self-interest ... that's pretty optimistic on your part.

Footnotes:
1 National Coalition on Health Care website
2 Public Citizen, April 18, 2002
3 Public Citizen, April 18, 2002
4 Fillon, p 77
5 Fillon, p 178
6 Mercola.com
7 FDA website
8 Fillon, p 144
9 Walker, p 230
10 Goldberg, p 51
11 Gaby, p 249
12 Kassirer, p 91
13 Goldberg, p 73

17 - The Drug Companies: Business v. Health

The medication marketplace is incredibly competitive. You have monster corporations like Novartis, Merck, Parke-Davis, Pfizer, SmithKline Beecham, Takeda, Bayer, Aventis, Eli Lilly, & Searle, to name a few. In these companies, doctors don't make the final decisions. Businesspeople make them. Marketing people make them. To sustain monster corporations requires monster income, and that requires outstanding marketing.

Meanwhile, the sharks are always circling, looking for any sign of weakness. Like, for instance, pulling a drug off the shelves because of a few deaths here and there. How could you possibly have worse publicity than admitting that your products kill people?

The pharmaceutical companies spend way more on ads than they spend in product research and development.[1]

How do you suppose drug company execs – businesspeople – react to rising rates of obesity or diabetes? Yes, it means heartbreak for millions more people. But the execs also know that it's increasing their market size, their company bottom line, and their personal bonuses.

Remember Chapter 2, about Merck & patents & statin drugs & CoQ10 depletion? What does someone do when there's a conflict between *your* interest and a drug being marketed by *their* company? Put yourself in their place. Do they safeguard you? Or do they safeguard their company, family, job, friends, salary, prestige, new car, country club membership, their future, & their retirement?

Inventing Diseases And Creating Markets

Selling cures for imaginary diseases is where the drug industry really rakes in the cash. Real need barely enters the picture. TV ads transform normal body changes to life-threatening disfigurement with only one solution – some new wonder drug.

It has always been true that as men age, they use the bathroom more at night. No big deal. Drug manufacturers saw an opportunity, and nighttime bathroom trips became a disease. They concocted TV commercials to convince doctors & patients that drug treatment was required.

To create 'new' disease, drug companies will:

1. Find a university professor. Fund him to write a book, or to do a media tour around the U.S.
2. Hire a sports celebrity or actor to meet with journalists, and to attend public forums, to create the need.

You'll notice also one obvious standard marketing practice: choose your market first, then develop a product. And the market they are all choosing is upscale Americans with the money & insurance to pay for expensive drugs. They divide that market into

1. toenail fungus sufferers
2. worried "multi-nighttime bathroom trips" people
3. bad hair day victims
4. embarrassed bedwetters
5. etc., etc., etc.

Then TV ads portray normal everyday ups and downs as a new disease in need of drug treatment. Invented diseases include:

- male pattern baldness
- wrinkles
- toenail fungus
- pre-hypertension
- bedwetting
- unwanted facial hair
- erectile dysfunction
- persistent sadness
- shyness

The really big money is in taking risk factors for future possible diseases and turning them into a drug treatment. So the focus is on obesity, cholesterol or high blood pressure. Huge markets for each. To build demand for their products and services, companies sponsor awareness-raising campaigns to make common unwanted (but normal) conditions look as severe and widespread as possible.

Redefining Old Diseases

Large companies, fiercely fighting for customers, constantly expand the definition of depression to increase the numbers who need treatment. After the 9/11 terrorist attack, they advertised "post-traumatic stress disorder" treatments.

Eli Lilly, facing the end of its patented blockbuster, Prozac™, recently relaunched the famous drug with a fancy new pink makeover and a new name – Sarafem™. This "Prozac™ in Pink" is now marketed to women as a treatment for severe PMS. And that PMS, by the way, has evolved to PMDD – Pre-Menstrual Dysphoric Disorder

Drug giant GlaxoSmithKline has taken paroxetine (Paxil™ in North America) and had it approved to treat what we used to call social phobia or shyness.

Where are all the new wonder drugs to cure the awful REAL diseases that have plagued us for so long? Guess the research team is working on it. They'll no doubt show up some day. Meanwhile, relax & take your Sarafem™.

Targeting Healthy People

Healthy people are a largely untapped market for the drug companies. Can you picture the marketing sessions where they brainstorm how to get into the "worried well"?

You've probably seen ads using celebrities to change public thinking about sexual difficulties, stomach problems, etc. Brokers match up celebrities & drug companies. People trust celebrities – that's why they're effective in drug ads. But the fact is, they're on the drug company payroll.

Disease prevention in healthy people with so-called "risk factors" like high blood pressure or high cholesterol is lucrative. Drug companies have redefined these measurable markers to encompass vast numbers of healthy people.

For instance: drug companies support patient groups like the National High Blood Pressure Education Program in the US. In 2003, the group announced a new warning about "pre-hypertension", which ratcheted down the definition of high blood pressure from 140 over 90 to 120 over 80. So overnight, millions of healthy people suddenly became medication-needing patients.[2]

Statins are now prescribed for healthy people as a preventative. The American Diabetes Association has recommended that all diabetics start statins, in case some benefit is someday discovered! Statins cause dangerous side effects. They lower cholesterol by interfering with liver function. It's not something to mess with. You can easily wind up with new symptoms or disorders, go to your doctor, and get diagnosed with another disease. Result? Another prescription drug, and more nutrient deficiencies.

It's called "upselling" - getting the same customer to buy more stuff, increasing your profit margin. Perfect business model for office supplies, maybe. Not so good for your health, however. As you recognize what the drug companies do in their marketing, how comfortable do you feel letting them make your health care decisions for you?

Research v. Marketing

The Pharmaceutical Research and Manufacturers Association (PhRMA) reports that, since 1995, R&D staff of US brand-name drug companies have decreased by 2%, while marketing staff have increased by 59%. Currently, 22% of staff are employed in R&D, while 39% are in marketing.[3]

As an old mentor used to tell me, pay attention to what a person pays attention to, and you'll know what their intentions are.

Drugs v. Nutrition

The way a pharmaceutical company can make lots of money is by developing medications that can be patented. Natural herbs and foods as well as medications that can no longer be patented won't be "pushed" in advertising because there's no real money to be made on them.[4] Could this explain why none of our players – drug companies, doctors, academia, the media, the FDA – seem to have any interest whatsoever in nutrition ... other than to legally regulate it?

Footnotes
1 Tracy, p 43
2 Cassels
3 Socolar
4 Long, p 11

18 - The FDA – Politics & Conflicts of Interest

Airplanes are built, licensed and flown according to standards set by the Federal Aviation Administration (FAA). But when there's a crash, the National Transportation Safety Board, (NTSB) investigates & recommends changes. Why? Because the FAA would have a conflict of interest investigating crashes of planes it approved & licensed.

But the FDA approves pharmaceuticals AND investigates injuries & deaths caused by those pharmaceuticals. So to an extent, they are actually investigating themselves. And in so doing, they rely on the drug companies to provide data on deaths and illnesses caused by drug company products!

Is THAT the type of system you want to trust your health and your family's health to?

The FDA's Actual Power Is Limited

They can request compliance. They send 2 kinds of enforcement letters to police drug company conduct. If a company refuses to comply, the FDA can't impose fines or other punishments. They must go through the courts for an injunction. So there is no compelling reason for a drug company to comply with an FDA letter.

When an FDA safety team identifies a problem drug, it evaluates a drug's riskiness and recommends what the FDA should do. Then that paperwork is sent to the review team that actually approved the drug in the first place. They analyze the drug's benefits, talk with the manufacturer, and help decide whether or not to withdraw approval for the drug.

So you have the same people who approved the drug now responsible for saying, "Whoops! We made a mistake." How often is THAT going to happen?

Since the drug companies pay the FDA for each drug approved, what happens when an FDA reviewer recommends against approving a "bad" drug? In some cases, the FDA removes the employee! The following comes from *The Los Angeles Times* of December 6, 1998:

Rezulin, a diabetes drug, was launched in March, 1997 by Warner-Lambert Co. Within months, it had been linked to at least 33 deaths due to liver failure. The drug was withdrawn in Britain. But the FDA left it on the market in the US.

What did the FDA do? **One medical officer who opposed Rezulin's approval was removed as the chief reviewer of the drug.** *Two other FDA physicians who recommended approval conceded in interviews that the agency initially overlooked compelling evidence of Rezulin's danger to the liver.*

The FDA decision to approve Rezulin without at least recommending that patients undergo precautionary liver testing "was an enormous blunder," said Dr. Curt D. Furberg, a drug testing specialist and head of public health sciences at Wake Forest University. "It's amazing that Rezulin is still on the market."[1]

The FDA is surely overwhelmed. And Congress keeps pushing for more & faster drug approvals, to satisfy their contributors & interest group pressure. Result? **The drug industry correctly believes it can get away with more violative advertising than ever.**[2]

A study of prescription drug ads showed "many claims prove to be inaccurate or misleading." (published

June 1,1992, in the *Annals of Internal Medicine*.) Medical experts reviewed 109 ads from the country's ten leading medical journals. Using the FDA's guidelines for pharmaceutical company ads, **the reviewers "indicated that 92% of advertisements were not in compliance in at least one area" of the FDA's guidelines.** Conclusion? The FDA is unable or unwilling to enforce its rules on drug advertising.[3]

So ... are the FDA bureaucrats owned by the politicians? Or do they stake out positions and then can't admit to being wrong? Or are they just totally overwhelmed by lack of money & personnel? Take your choice.

How FDA Personnel Is Assigned

- "The FDA's drug-marketing enforcement office has only 40 employees to review more than 30,000 pieces of promotional material a year. Those include TV and print ads, sales brochures for doctors and company postings on Internet sites."[4]
- The FDA does not get even one dollar to track whether all these new drugs are safe. So approvals are way up, and safety is way down:
- FDA personnel assigned to process new drug applications: 1,300 employees. One drug company alone – Pfizer – has 4,500 people in its sales force.[6]
- FDA personnel who track whether drugs are hurting people: 72 employees (including only 13 with formal epidemiology training – the science of spotting medical disasters.[5]

So new drugs & massive advertising bring big sales quicker than ever ... and bad drugs create more damage quicker. The FDA's current 72-person safety team uses tools designed when speed wasn't so important. They're overwhelmed. Mostly, they wait for bad news to come in. Meanwhile, drug company reps hover over the FDA approval teams, doing their best to speed up the process.

Funding

"Asking the FDA to rein in the pharmaceuticals industry is a bit like sending someone out to catch Niagara Falls in a bucket."[7] The drug companies have way more money. Law change has boomed the drug industry to a $$$ level the FDA can't come anywhere close to regulating:

- FDA's annual budget for approving, labeling, and monitoring drugs: $290 million
- FDA "safety team" budget for investigating problem drugs: $15 million
- Drug industry annual promotional budget: $11-12 Billion!
- So the total FDA budget is less than ¼ of 1% of the promotional budget of the drug companies!
- And the FDA "safety team" budget is about 1/100th of 1% of the drug company promotional budget!

The drug industry has a VERY loud voice, backed by a world of money. It's simple human nature to pay attention to what they say. The 1992 & 1997 law changes have elevated the drug industry financially above every other industry on the planet. Every year FDA goes to Congress for money to regulate the drug companies … who donate money to every member of Congress.

How can a 72-person FDA safety team monitor the effects of more than 13,000 prescription drugs on 200 million people with a budget of around $15 million a year?

A Few Interesting FDA Policies

▶ Ads cited for making too strong a claim just add the line, "individual results may vary" – and they've been approved to go back on the air.

▶ Advertised drugs may be FDA-approved – but the FDA only requires clinical testing of as few as 1,000 people.[8] If this drug kills one in every 2,000, ... oh, well. Maybe you'll get lucky. Even if a new drug is safe, it may not be any better than older, cheaper stuff that's gone generic.

▶ Drug ads and free samples usually decide which drug doctors treat patients with. Ads are ads. You find a ton of them in the mass consumer magazines. They exaggerate a drug's benefits, then downplay the hazards. "And since the FDA screens only 10% - 20% of all drug promotions, physicians are forced to take drug companies at their word."[9]

▶ The FDA's job is to set & enforce standards for drug ads. Yet, according to a University of California study published in *The Wall Street Journal*, 60% of the pharmaceutical ads from medical journals violated FDA guidelines. But the FDA has done nothing about these violations.[10]

Footnotes
1 – Wellman
2 – Wolfe, p 10
3 – Glenmullen, p 232
4 – Schmit
5 – Pomper
6 – Morrison
7 – Pomper
8 – FDA website
9 – Feuer, p 73
10 – Goldberg, p 48

19 - Some Pretty Bad Doctoring

You probably assume your doctor protects you from unsafe drugs. But "unsafe" doesn't stop drug companies from pushing doctors to prescribe. In January, 1997, the FDA fast-tracked Parke-Davis' diabetes drug Rezulin™, approving it with just 6 months' testing. Users started dying. Britain revoked Rezulin™ approval.

But not here in the U.S. Even though FDA epidemiologist David J. Graham told an FDA advisory board that anyone taking Rezulin™ risked sudden liver failure, the drug was not withdrawn. Similar drugs were available that didn't kill anyone. So why would a doctor still prescribe Rezulin™?

Here's one possible answer: in spring 1999, Parke-Davis invited New York area doctors to a "special scientific lecture" at "the Club Bar and Grille ... Madison Square Garden." After a short lecture & dinner, the doctors were taken to their courtside seats for the New York Knicks -. Toronto Raptors basketball game.[1]

Doctors Are Human

What doctor will admit to being influenced by drug company money? Probably none. But the drug industry spends $18 billion a year and a lot of time learning how to push doctors' buttons. They get their money's worth.

The drug companies don't need to look into a doctor's soul. They have better tools. For instance, drug companies & their reps can just subscribe to the IMS Health database (**http://www.imshealth.com**) **to see exactly what prescriptions each doctor writes!**

Armed with THAT information, they know exactly who to target for any drug. The computer spits out a marketing list of the exact doctors they should invite to a weekend retreat in the Bahamas for a two-hour symposium about a new product.

Even the *Journal of the American Medical Association* (*"Is a Gift Ever Just a Gift?"*, Vol. 283 No. 3, January 19, 2000) concluded that drug company sales kits influence prescriptions, including "non-rational" prescribing.[2]

Drug companies spend $5 billion a year just sending sales reps to doctors' offices. Doctors get a steady stream of drug company reps in their office. And of the 90,000 drug reps in the US, many are beautiful, young former college cheerleaders. (Most doctors are still male.) There's now even an employment agency in Memphis that matches up former college cheerleaders with pharmaceutical companies.[3]

And if the reps need any other advantage, they can read the scouting reports in the IMS Health database. If Doc goes to a conference, the young ladies are there, too. And Doc gets free journals from all the drug companies. Do you think all this has an effect on doctors' thinking & decisions?

Drug companies spend over $18 billion a year just promoting their products to physicians. With about 600,000 doctors in active practice, that's over $30,000 per doctor![4]

Almost everything doctors and consumers know about medications comes from drug companies. The drug companies write & distribute package inserts, drug ads, and the doctors' Bible, the *Physicians' Desk Reference*. Need medication and dosage info? Most doctors look it up in the PDR. Or they ask a drug company rep (easy to find, since they're in the doctors' offices every day). Or they check the medical journal product ads. Result? Your health pretty much depends on the drug companies always doing the right thing.[5]

It takes time to speak to a patient about exercise, weight control, and diet. It takes less time to just write a prescription. How many doctors choose the easier course?

Doctors will tell you they're professional, that they're not influenced by the advertising, the gifts, the cheerleaders, the trips, the personal attention, etc. What do YOU think?

Is Your Body The Same As Your Neighbor's?

Many doctors prescribe the same number of milligrams for all patients, despite different ages & conditions. It's called "standard dosing." But the fact is, the numbers in your blood test results are different from everybody else's. Too high a dose in the wrong person can be deadly. People metabolize drugs differently.

Lower doses are often just as effective. But manufacturers want quick approval for new drugs, and testing to determine the lowest effective amount takes time. So doctors will often prescribe the same dose for every patient. That practice is absolutely not in YOUR best interest.

Patients hear about new drugs before their doctors do. It's not unusual for consumers to ask their doctor for prescription drugs that the doctor knows little or nothing about. Studies show that if you ask your doctor to prescribe a specific drug, you have better than a 75% chance that he will do so. TV & magazine ads teach people how to describe their symptoms so they'll get a certain medication.

Medical Graft

In 1990, the FDA forbid "gifts of substantial value" to doctors. So the drug companies shifted from giving stereos & fax machines to dinners & cruises & baseball games. To read all about medical graft, go to **http://nofreelunch.org**, a website dedicated to spotlighting & getting rid of the problem.

Drug reps regularly offer to take the clinic staff to lunch. Nurses & doctor assistants have doctors' ears … and keys to the sample closets that reps can stock. Reps give out a ton of promotions: pens, pads, small toys with the company's logo. It's simple psychology. All these freebies build up a mental debt.

Here's the thinking on free samples. Doc gives drug samples to Sue, who feels gratitude to Doc … who feels gratitude to the drug company. It's easy to see how a doctor is more inclined to prescribe the medicine and the patient more inclined to ask for it.

Some salesmen tell of out-right extortion by doctors. ("I won't prescribe your product unless you get us on a Caribbean cruise.")[6]

Put 'Em On The Payroll!

Really buy Doc's loyalty. Get Doc on the company payroll. Then they'll REALLY do some prescribing!

In winter of 1999, to promote Celebrex, Searle invited 300 doctors & pharmacists to an Orlando getaway.

Searle used the IMS database (**http://www.imshealth.com**) to target real opinion leaders. In Orlando, the guests were recruited to a national "speakers bureau."". Searle paid $500 each for coming to Florida and $500 for each speech they gave on Celebrex™ after returning home. Not to mention the trip itself ... all-you-could-eat gourmet food, an open bar, & exclusive group use of Universal Studios theme park for the evening.[7]

PS – Celebrex™ broke all 1st year records, bringing Searle about $1 Billion in its first year out. Because it was an enormous scientific breakthrough? Not exactly. Celebrex™ is a painkiller, like aspirin, acetaminophen, and ibuprofen, but different. Some tests showed it was less effective.[8]

One rep let his targets win phony contests (like guessing the number of pills in a jar). Then, he'd find out their hot button. Booze. No problem. Women? He had phone numbers ready. Drugs? Absolutely. A lot of docs like codeine-laced Tylenol IV™ (liquid formula) in their cocktails.[9]

The Hippocratic Oath – New & Improved!

A recent study in *Health Affairs* magazine ("How Medical Marketing Influences Doctors and Patients" by Ben Harder) reported that 76% of the respondents who saw a drug on TV and asked their doctors for it were successful. Few doctors argue with a patient's prescription preferences unless they know it's a medication that will hurt him. The commercials are like an "upsell", bringing more money to the doctor's bottom line.

Not only are we an overmedicated society, we are a self-medicated one. Doctors prescribe more drugs than ever before AND the American public is buying more over-the-counter medications than ever.[10]

83

"Each year, hundreds of thousands of Americans who are actually suffering from common medical conditions such as hyperthyroidism, Lyme disease, and even poor nutrition are misdiagnosed with psychiatric disorders. Studies show that the rate of misdiagnosis is more than 4 in 10."[11]

Doctors aren't required to report bad drug reactions, so they usually don't. Drug companies must report adverse events, but they get most of their information from doctors. Estimates are only 1-10 % of adverse drug events ever get reported.[12]

So how many misdiagnosed patients get prescriptions? Whatever the number, every single one of them causes further nutrient depletion. Putting your health in the hands of our medical system seems a lot like Russian roulette.

Footnotes
1 – Pomper
2 – JAMA
3 – Saul
4 – Kassirer, p 78
5 – Cohen, p 16
6 – Pomper
7 – Pomper
8 – Pomper
9 – Kippen
10 – Strand, p 169
11 – Walker, p 230
12 – Pomper

20 - Scientists: The Academic - Industrial Complex

It's been 50 years since President Eisenhower coined the phrase, "Military-Industrial Complex." Ike was warning the public of the natural conflict of interest when the military and business got together. The military needed business to develop & produce lots of shiny new war toys. Business needed the U.S. military because no entity in the world had deeper pockets.

Academia constantly talked about and wrote about the Military-Industrial Complex. Professors from coast to coast were up in arms about the terrible conflux of military (public) money and industrial arms production. They saw nothing but evil coming from this joint venture.

Many still think the same thing today. But today, we have perhaps a greater, more immediate threat to our lives: The Academic-Industrial Complex.

Question: What the difference between a scientist and a prostitute?

Answer: A prostitute only screws one person at a time.

Conflict of Interest?

That's not all. Consider industry-funded research & training.

On one side, you have students. What they want is financial grants. To get them, they need to get published. On the other side, you have companies. They have a ton of money burning a hole in their pocket. What they want is scholarly studies to make their products look good. It's a marriage made in heaven.

Is it any wonder that industry funding for academic research octupled between 1980 and 1997, as research costs climbed, and the rate of growth of federal support declined?[1]

A study of major engineering research centers found that 35% admitted they would allow corporate sponsors to delete information from papers prior to publication.

In 1997, Sheldon Krimsky (professor of public policy at Tufts University) surveyed 61,134 articles in 181 journals. A quarter of the biomedical researchers at the time were receiving funding from industry. But only 0.5 percent disclosed a conflict of interest related to the topic of the article.[2]

Conflicts of interest? Judge for yourself:
1. Professors get paid by companies for their research. They often hold stock or have other financial ties to the companies paying them.
2. Universities invest in these companies.
3. Regular publication delays of more than 30-60 days and other editorial constraints protect a discovery owed to a corporate interest.
4. Professors abide by proprietary restrictions on basic research tools.
5. Professors tailor the research agenda to the desires of the company.

Even without sponsors, most drug studies are favorable. Unsponsored research papers are 79% positive on the drug in question; it's 98% positive on industry-sponsored research. Most medical journals publish sponsored research, with disclosure.[3]

What happens to *negative* reviews? "Some researchers who have tried to publish unflattering findings have been threatened with lawsuits."[4]

A 2003 study found that nearly half of medical school faculty, who serve on Institutional Review Boards (IRB) to advise on clinical trial research, also serve as consultants to the pharmaceutical industry.[5]

Impure Science - The Symposium Circuit

"More than 60% of clinical studies ... published in scientific journals like *Nature* and *The New England Journal of Medicine* ... are increasingly likely to be designed, controlled, and sometimes even ghost-written by marketing departments, rather than academic scientists."[6]

Publish a couple favorable papers, and you may go out on the symposium circuit. When Dr. Michael Gorback was on Duke Medical School faculty, Smith Kline asked him to do a presentation on Smith Kline's antacid Tagamet™. Dr. Gorback was given a complete lecture script & slides. He had his own ideas but Smith Kline flew him to Boston for a rehearsal. Another professor there was perfectly OK with a script he hadn't even read.[8]

Symposium papers get leveraged. They're reprinted in bound "supplements" to medical journals (same font, so they look like journal articles). Drug reps give the supplements to doctors, hoping they'll pass for research papers.

Let's say you're a young PhD. I own a pharmaceutical company. I hire you, 45 grand a year, and say, "Look. We're going to experiment on the toxic levels of this formula. Here

87

are the results we need for FDA approval. Here's your lab coat. There's your room."

THAT is "science" these days!

Footnotes:
1 - Press & Washburn
2 - Brownlee
3 - Cho
4 - Pomper
5 - Null, p 10
6 - Brownlee
7 - Pomper

21 - Turn On The TV, Relax, And Take Your Pills

Philosophers through the ages have told us that we become what we think about. Well, if you're watching TV 4 hours a day and you see 25 ads a day, 7 days a week, telling you that you might be sick with this or that or the other thing – many of them invented diseases – what kind of effect does that have on you?

Our health is being sold to us like soap.

Ad agencies, drug companies, and the major television networks lobbied for less restrictive rules, and, in August 1997, the FDA issued a "clarification" of its 30-year-old regulations. Television commercials may now name both the product and the disease, as long as viewers are given information about "major" risks of the drug and directed to other sources of information - websites, magazine ads, toll-free numbers - for more detail.

A recent study in the *Journal of General Internal Medicine* found that nearly half of respondents believed that drug ads are prescreened and somehow sanctioned by the FDA. Did you know that the FDA is forbidden by law from requiring advertising preclearance? All the FDA can require is that a copy be sent to its office when the ad begins to air.[1]

The media have a double standard. They're happy to use video news releases from the pharmaceutical and medical technology industry. Morning talk shows are full of medical technology miracles and wonder drugs, using the drug company videos. Plus, of course; page after page of drug ads in the print media. For example, Pfizer purchased all of the advertising space in an entire issue of *Time* magazine on the "Future of Medicine." Johnson & Johnson bought the ad space of an entire issue of *Newsweek*.[2]

When a major advertising benefactor like Pfizer releases new drugs, how fired-up do you think *Time* magazine gets about searching for any problems with those drugs?

Does Advertising Work?

Schering-Plough launched Claritin's[TM] war against sneezing in 1998 with $185 million in TV ads. Sales more than doubled to $2.1 billion. Pfizer spent $57 million on Zyrtec[TM] TV ads in 1999. Result? Sales up 32%. Aventis spent $43 million promoting Allegra[TM] ... sales up 50%. [3]

Scott-Levin, a pharmaceutical consulting company in Pennsylvania, says that doctor visits by patients claiming allergy symptoms were stable from 1990 – 1998: 13 to 14 million a year. In 1999, allergy visits spiked to 18 million allergy visits. Do TV ads work? You betcha![4]

Some health plans spend more on prescription drugs than on in-patient hospitalization. Why? TV advertising.

Some drug commercial budgets rival TV shows and movies. Why not? If you're paying next to nothing for raw materials, and then you can turn around and charge $50 or $150 or $500 or $????, then you have a margin that allows a lot of big-budget advertising.

Drug company PR firms hire freelance medical journalists to write articles and submit them to unsuspecting medical journals. Healthcare PR firms also move fast to "squash" any negative news about their clients, or to promote damaging news about others.[5]

The average number of prescriptions per person in the US increased from 7.3 in 1992 to 10.4 in 2000. And today we buy more expensive medications, because those are the ones you see on TV. From 1999-2000, prescriptions for the 50 most heavily advertised drugs rose six times faster than prescriptions for all other drugs, according to Katharine Greider's book, *The Big Fix*.[6]

TV As Your Doctor

So patients direct their own treatment based on TV commercials. Antidepressants come with handy checklists of symptoms. Everything is a disease, and not only is it a disease, but it's a disease that you can get a pill for. Result? People wind up pressing their doctors for a powerful drug they don't really need.

Prescription drugs now are treated like any consumer product – laundry detergent, cereal, cars, furniture wax. You get a catchy tune, smiling faces, big promises. If you buy oatmeal, you probably won't do yourself too much damage. But when you see a commercial and then go to your doctor to get some powerful prescription drug, you risk serious illness and even death. And that's BEFORE you calculate the damage done to your body by nutrient depletion.

Advertorials

An advertising tactic of long-standing use is the advertorial. Rather than looking like an ad, the advertorial looks just like the news or editorial comments in a publication. It's written in columns, often using the same font. Done correctly, an advertorial gets more credibility than the regular run of ads. It's an effective method of advertising.

The drug companies have adapted this technique to their own purposes. They distribute a collection of advertorials to doctors' offices, designed to look like excerpts from some professional symposiuim. In reality, it's ad copy written by professionals. Misleading headings make the reader think he's reading selected summaries of key talks from the conference. Somewhere in the publication, there's always a disclaimer that these comments don't come from the actual conference. But it's in small print, and is often overlooked.

Footnotes:
1 - Belkin
2 - Morrison, page 79
3 - Belkin
4 - Belkin
5 - Fillon, page 146
6 – Fillon

22 – Are You Skeptical?
Some Questions For You

If you're skeptical of what you've read, I understand.

On the one side, you've got the doctors, the drug companies, the universities, the government, and the never-ending media messages. On the other side, there are a few voices in the wilderness like this book. I can hear your somewhat ironic question now: "So you're saying YOU are right and EVERYBODY ELSE is wrong?"

Yes. That is what I'm saying.

Some questions to help bring this all into focus:

- Vioxx^{TM} is Merck's anti-arthritis drug. It killed & injured people and has generated over 4,000 lawsuits. There may be a lot more. Because drugs kill, lawsuits are common in this business. So how much do you want to rely on information given out by spokesmen for the drug companies & doctors who may be subject to those lawsuits? Common sense says that what they tell you is geared to minimize their liability. What do you think?

- If you believe "germs" cause disease, how can you explain our survival up until the 21st century? Bacteria & viruses are the oldest and toughest life forms. Why didn't they kill us off thousands of years ago, when we didn't have antibiotics and all the hi-tech drugs you see on TV. Why are we still alive?

- Why did Merck get Patents No. 4929437 and 4933165 in 1990 ... and never use them?

- Why does the Canadian government advise statin drug users of the need to supplement ... while in the U.S., the FDA does not?

- Why aren't people getting healthier with all these "lifesaving" drugs?

- Does it make sense that life-altering drugs with sometimes fatal side effects are marketed direct to the consumer on TV along with cereal and laundry soap?

- We couldn't trust the celebrities, the doctors, the manufacturers, the media, the scientists, or the government regulators from the 1920s through the 1960s, when they all told us how wonderful cigarettes were. And now they're all on the drug bandwagon. Doesn't it make you wonder?

- Are you aware that NO drug ever treats the *cause* of a physical problem ... only the *symptoms*?

- The problem your body has is nutritional. Why would you think the solution is pharmaceutical?

- Did you know that the reason drugs make you feel great is that they block your metabolic pathways – stopping the communication of pain – without ever addressing or even knowing the *source* of the pain?

- Have you read in the mainstream media how the over-prescribing of antibiotics has lead to a generation of superbugs, that no drug will kill?

94

- Does a drug move your body closer to, or further away from, normal function?

- According to the *Journal of the American Medical Association* (JAMA) of April 14, 1998, "Adverse drug reactions are the fourth leading cause of death in America." Does THAT sound like a "wonder cure?"

- Do you believe the FDA safety division – the ones responsible for spotting dangerous prescription drugs – can be effective with a budget $1/100^{th}$ of 1% the size of the drug companies' promotional budget?

- Many doctors use "standard dosing," prescribing the same amount of drug to every patient, no matter how different their test results. Is your body the same as your neighbor's? Does this sound like someone who's really looking out for your best interest?

- Has ANY doctor ever suggested that you supplement your prescription with nutrients to avoid depletion?

- You KNOW your body needs water to get rid of toxins. Why do so many doctors prescribe diuretics to purge fluid from your body? What happens to the toxins that can't be removed when your fluid levels are down? Where do they go?

- Every year the FDA goes to Congress for money to regulate the drug companies ... who donate money to every member of Congress. Does this concern you?

- Does it make sense to you that medical journal product evaluations are often written by someone being paid by the company that makes the product?

23 – Pin The Tail
On The Donkey

"Adverse drug reactions are the fourth leading cause of death in America. Reactions to prescription and over-the-counter medications kill far more people annually than all illegal drug use combined." – *Journal of the American Medical Association*

It's important to understand the principles of your body's workings, and its breakdowns. You need to know when to call the towtruck, and when to get under the hood yourself.

Truth #1 is very simple and obvious:

**Nutrients are the building blocks
your body uses for a healthy system.**

Truth #2 is also simple & obvious:

**Prescription and over-the-counter drugs are
extraneous chemicals, not nutrients (i.e., your
body will never have a Tylenol^{TM} deficiency).**

Truth #3 is also simple & obvious:

**The scientists formulate a drug to alter a single
biochemical process in your system, in order to
change the level of a single marker that is
considered out of sync (e.g., cholesterol level, blood-
sugar level, arterial plaque, homocysteine level, etc.)**

Truth #4 is simple, maybe not-so-obvious, but truly crucial:

Any drug you take is *systemic*, not targeted. It will hinder MANY biochemical processes in your body. In so doing, it causes nutrient deficiencies.

In fact, drugs are actually ANTI-nutrients. Let's review some other main points:

1. In every TV commercial you see for every drug you take, they talk about "side effects." What causes side effects is that every drug you take depletes nutrients in your body. Problem is, many side effects take months or years to become full-fledged problems. You'll never connect them to that drug.

2. Every drug company KNOWS their products deplete nutrients, but they don't tell you that. In Canada, makers of statin drugs are required by law to tell you that their product depletes Co-enzyme Q10. Not in the U.S. So they don't say a word. Does that sound like they have your best interest at heart?

3. The FDA does not require ANY testing of new drugs for causing nutrient deficiencies. Does that sound like YOUR health is a big concern to them?

4. Doctors focus on disease. Most don't understand what causes health. Most don't know much, if anything, about nutrition. For many, most of their ongoing education comes from drug company publications. Not to mention some of their ongoing income.

5. Scientists get paid big bucks to write papers favorable to particular drugs. When they write something unfavorable, they are out of work.

6. Politicians from both parties get major contributions from drug companies.

7. The mass media combine to take in billions of dollars of profit each year from drug company ads.

Every one of these players would suffer financially if you cut down your drug purchases. If you want to trust in them, that's your choice. Just recognize that each of them has a conflict of interest when they advise you.

Of course, I'm a strong believer that you need nutrients, not drugs. And I sell a full-spectrum, nutrient-dense nutritional product. That's also a conflict of interest. Consider that as you decide what to do. You need to decide where you see truth, and what it means to your future. If you put your faith in the pharmaceutical path, you are almost certainly decreasing your life expectancy.

I can't tell you how many people have told me, "Well, so what? Everybody's gotta die of something!"

Yes they do. But they DO NOT have to spend the last 5 or 10 or 15 or 20 years of their life in constant degeneration and increasing disability due to nutrient deficiency. That's a condition that American society has pioneered over the last 50 years. You've probably seen some friend or family member suffer that way. Nobody in their right mind wants that.

Truth is truth. It doesn't matter whether you like it or not. Or if it fits your plans, or disrupts your life, or if it 100% changes everything you're doing. Once you've read these ideas, no matter how long you live, you'll NEVER get them out of your mind. If you continue on that pharmaceutical path, you WILL get sicker.

It's YOUR Responsibility

No way can your doctor – or ANY doctor – know everything. They have too much to do. I'll bet they don't even learn 5% of the new stuff in their own field, let alone something completely new to them like nutrition. It's NOT your doctor's fault. But it's YOUR health. You need to take an active stance. Do some research. There are many good books on the subject now. Check out the publications in the bibliography. Do some online searches.

Your doctor, your pharmacist, the drug companies, the FDA, the scientists, the media … none of them are going to pay your medical expenses. You need to take control of your family's health and make some tough choices. You need to be skeptical about the claims being made about drugs and disease, about the labels attached to them, and the conditions they're being told they have.

Bottom line is, you need to pin the tail on the donkey. All our players have worked together to blindfold you and spin you around, hoping you'll totter off in the wrong direction like almost everybody else does.

But you've got the advantage now. You've gotten a peek through the blindfold. You know where the donkey is, and you sure as heck know where its butt is.

Go ahead. Stick that tail where it belongs. Your health and your family's health depend on it.

24 – A Word About Nutrition

I'm not suggesting you don't use prescription medications. There is a role for prescription medications, for antibiotics, heart medications, etc.

But there is absolutely NO QUESTION you need nutritional supplements, to replace the nutrients you've depleted by taking prescription drugs. You require nutrients as part of your treatment profile, to replace what is being destroyed.

There was a time when you got all the nutrients you need from a balanced diet. But modern farming has strip-mined our soils of nutrients. A pound of spinach today has 60% less nutrients than a pound of spinach did 40 years ago.

Look at the science. Everybody has a horrible diet. Heart disease is still the #1 killer in the U.S. And a key part of that is oxidative damage. So what is oxidation?

Simple. It's aging. It's rust. If you leave a nail outside, what happens? It rusts. It's exposed to environmental stress, heat stress, cold stress, moisture, pollution, etc.

Now put that nail in your home. Controlled temperature, controlled environment, controlled humidity. It won't rust as fast. **That is exactly what vitamins, minerals and other nutrients are – a protective environment for your body.**

Will the nail still rust? Yes. In 20 or 25 years, against 2 or 3 years if you leave it outside. That's oxidation, our greatest killer today.

As kids, then teenagers, then young adults ... where do we eat our meals? Burger King, McDonald's, Pizza Hut, Taco Bell. You absolutely don't get the right nutrients in your food. Over time, the oxidative damage and stress in your body is so devastating and so debilitating, disease begins.

Your body starts to break down. And then .. at 30, 40, 50 years of age ... you add on prescription drugs for diabetes, for blood pressure, for cholesterol. You go into atrial fibrillation.

Why does this happen to us? Why do you go into atrial fibrillation? Why do you get an irregular heartbeat? It's not just that you're getting old. It's because your body is starting to break down. Instead of going in the expected line, it starts to take a different road. The road becomes very circuitous, very dangerous.

Result? You end up using more energy to get from point A to point B. Your engine is not running efficiently. So just to get the same result you got a few years ago, you have to burn a lot more fuel. You burn a lot more nutrients.

So my questions for you are:
1. Are you taking any prescription medications?
2. Did you eat 6 or 8 servings of fruits & vegetables yesterday, as per the recommendation of the American Heart Association & the American Cancer Society?
3. Do you exercise at least 3-4 times a week?
4. Are you getting 8 hours sound sleep a night?
5. Are you drinking at least 8 glasses of water a day?

Consider your answers. If you take prescription meds, or if you don't eat all your fruits & veggies or exercise regularly or get your 8 hours sleep or drink your 8 glasses of water, then you absolutely need to be taking nutrients that your body doesn't break down & deplete.

I have personally used hundreds of nutritional products over the years. The all-time best nutrient source is ocean-based vegetation from a 100% pollution-free area. My favorite source of these sea nutrients is listed in the **"Recommended Vendors"** section. I strongly encourage you to try it.

25 – Why I Wrote This Book

September 26, 1989

Cheryl & I sat in shock in the doctor's office at Miami Children's Hospital, learning that our 4-year-old son Garth had Duchenne Muscular Dystrophy. The doctor sent us home with our misery and a brochure.

I won't go into the details of all the things I have seen wrong with our medical system since that date. There are plenty. I'll just mention two:

1. Maybe the most often-used treatment for Duchenne MD is the steroid prednizone. It offers no hope long-term and has awful short-term side effects, yet many parents opt for prednizone out of frustration that there's just nothing else to do.

2. Only boys get DMD. It's a genetic, inherited disease, passed from mother (the carrier) to son (the sufferer). Yet we had no history of DMD in the family. How could it be inherited? I've spoken to parents of over 100 other DMD boys through the years, and at least half will tell you the same thing ... no family history of DMD.

When you ask the doctors about this, they say, "Must be spontaneous mutation." So DMD is an inherited disease, but half the cases are "spontaneous mutation?"

Nuts! These doctors don't have a clue. When you don't understand the problem, you have no hope of a solution.

January 27, 1996

My mother finally died. She retired from IBM in 1984, full of hopes, plans & expectations for her golden years. Within 6 months, she was diagnosed with jaw cancer.

She had 5 operations over the next 10 years. After the first, they were all cosmetic. It's tough to look great when you've lost a jawbone. But Mom got worse with each surgery. And the doctors just kept operating, promising that the next round would restore her looks, and she could get on with her plans.

It never happened. Each surgery, she got worse, until she finally she was defeated and gave up the ghost. The four worthless surgeries destroyed the last 10 years of her life.

October 15, 1999

Cousin Bruce was my business partner & close friend. And he was hilarious. I laughed every day with Bruce around. I loved that guy!

Then out of the blue, the doctors gave him 2 years to live. They said they could only change that with surgery. They were right. They operated, and Bruce was dead in 6 weeks.

April 3, 2003

I lay in the hospital bed, looking up at the ceiling. The doctor told me the results of my cardiac catheterization: I did not have a blood vessel blockage. Instead, the reason my heartbeat had gone to 200 beats a minute was heart arrhythmia.

I knew about the arrhythmia, of course. I'd had it for years, maybe once every few weeks. Suddenly, I had a very bad episode and wound up in the hospital.

But it's what happened next that astonished me. I was discharged and given some prescriptions. And within a few weeks, my sporadic arrhythmia became DAILY arrhythmia! My heart condition was way worse.

And it stayed that way until a friend recommended a general nutritional supplement that might help. I began taking it, and there was an immediate lessening of both the frequency & the intensity of my arrhythmia.

Several months later, I added a 2nd supplement, designed specifically for heart problems. And within 3 months, my arrhythmia went away altogether! That has been an enormous change in my life.

So why did the arrhythmia disappear? Were my chronic lifetime nutrient deficiencies finally solved? I have no way of knowing for sure, but that certainly is what I think.

And I think the chances are very high that YOU also suffer from nutrient deficiencies, whether you see the symptoms yet or not. I highly recommend you do something about it.

Today

I have learned from experience not to trust the medical establishment. Because of that, I've done a lot of research into means of prevention of disease & bad health, rather than relying on the doctors to fix problems after they happen.

And today, the biggest threat I see comes from the fact that most people just accept what they're told by the drug companies, the doctors, the universities, and the media. (Nobody believes the politicians, but that's just one out of five!)

I hope you have found useful information in this book. I hope you are inspired to continue taking or to re-take responsibility for your family's health. If you do that, if you practice preventative medicine so that you don't become a victim of our prescription drug culture, then your health future is bright.

Bibliography

Abrahamson, John, "Overdosed America: The Broken Promise of American Medicine." HarperCollins, 2004. ISBN:: 0060568526

Cohen, Jay, MD, "Over Dose: The Case Against the Drug Companies: Prescription Drugs, Side Effects, and Your Health." Tarcher Putnam, New York, 2001

Cluff, Dr. Leighton F., "Controversies in Therapeutics." ed. Louis Lasagna, Saunders, 1980

Feuer, Elaine, "Innocent Casualties : The FDA's War Against Humanity." Dorrance Publishing Co, 1996. ISBN 0805938192

Fillon, Mike, "Ephedra Fact & Fiction: How Politics, the Press and Special Intrest Are Targeting You Rights to Vitamins, Minerals and Herbs." Woodland Publishing, 2004. ISBN: 1580543707

Gaby, Alan R., "Preventing and Reversing Osteoporosis." Prima Publishing, Rocklin, CA, 1994. ISBN: 0761500227

Glenmullen, Joseph, MD, "Prozac Backlash: Overcoming the Dangers of Prozac, Zoloft, Paxil, and Other Antidepressants with Safe, Effective Alternatives." Simon & Schuster, 2000. ISBN: 0-684-86001-5

Goldberg, Burton, "Alternative Medicine." Future Medicine Publishing, January 1997. ISBN:0963633430.

Greider, Katharine, The Big Fix: How the Pharmaceutical Industry Rips Off American Consumers. Public Affairs Books, 2003. ISBN: 1586481851

Kassirer, Jerome P., MD, "On the Take: How Medicine's Complicity with Big Business Can Endanger Your Health." Oxford University Press. New York, 2004. ISBN 0195300041

Long, Duncan, "Attaining Medical Self Sufficiency: An Informed Citizen's Guide, Sentinel Communications, Inc., 1-800-800-1865

McKeown, Thomas, "The Role of Medicine", Blackwell Scientific Publications, 1979

Morrison, Ian, "Health Care in the New Millennium: Vision, Values, and Leadership." Jossey-Bass Wiley Publishers, San Francisco. 2002. ISBN: 0-7879-6222-8

Pelton, Ross, RPh, PhD, CCN, and others, "The Drug-Induced Nutrient Depletion Handbook - 2nd Edition." Lexi Comp, 2001. ISBN 1-930598-45-9 591

Ruesch, Hans, "Naked Empress or The Great Medical Fraud." CIVIS Publications, Switzerland, 1982. ISBN 3-905280-02-7

Strand, Ray D., "Death by Prescription: The Shocking Truth Behind an Overmedicated Nation" Thomas Nelson Publishers, Nashville. ISBN: 0785264841

Tracy, Ann Blake, PhD., "PROZAC: PANACEA OR PANDORA? The Rest of the Story" on the New Class of SSRI Antidepressants." 1994. ISBN: 0-916095-59-2

Walker, Sydney MD, "A Dose of Sanity: Mind, Medicine, and Misdiagnosis." October, 1997, page 230 ISBN: 0-471-19262-7.

Wolfe, Sydney M., and others and Public Citizen's Health Research Group, "Worst Pills Best Pills." Pocket Books Health ISBN: 0-671-01918-X

Magazine Articles

Belkin, Lisa, "Prime Time Pushers", Mother Jones, March/April 2001 Issue
Brownlee, Shannon, "Doctors Without Borders: Why you can't trust medical journals anymore." Washington Monthly, April, 2004.
Cassels, Alan. "Peddling Paranoia," The New Internationalist, Nov, 2003.
Cho, M.K. and Bero, L. A. (1996) "The quality of drug studies published in symposium proceedings." Annals of Internal Medicine 124:485-489.
Friedman, Michael, "Efficient FDA Drug Review Benefits Cancer Patients, FDA Deputy Commissioner Michael Friedman, MD, Journal of American Medical Association (JAMA), on May 12, 1999.
Harder, Ben, "How Medical Marketing Influences Doctors and Patients." Health Affairs magazine.
http://flatrock.org.nz/topics/drugs/how_drug_companies_spin_doctors.htm
Moore, Thomas J. and others, "Time to Act on Drug Safety," JOURNAL OF THE AMERICAN MEDICAL ASSOCIATION Vol. 279, No. 19 (May 20, 1998), pgs. 1571-1573
Mundell, E. J., "Doctors Urge Cholesterol Drugs for Diabetics." HealthDay News April 19, 2004
Kippen A. "Doctored results: how drug companies bribe doctors and medical journals." Washington Monthly. October 1990:.38-42
Pomper, Stephen, "Drug Rush: Why the prescription drug market is unsafe at high speeds," The Washington Monthly, May 2000
Press, Eyal and Jennifer Washburn "The Kept University", The Atlantic Monthly, March 2000 | Volume 285 No. 3
http://www.mindfully.org/GE/The-Kept-UniversityMar00.htm
Public Citizen
Researchers John & Sonja McKinlay
Rutter, Virginia and Arma, Tom, "Who stole fertility?" Psychology Today. Mar/Apr 96.
Saul, Stephanie, "Gimme an Rx! Cheerleaders Pep Up Drug Sales," New York Times Nov. 28, 2005
Schmit, Julie, "FDA Races To Keep Up With Drug Ads That Go Too Far", USA Today, 5/30/2005
Socolar, Deborah, and Alan Sager, 'Pharmaceutical marketing and research spending: the evidence does not support PhRMA's claims', Boston University School of Public Health. a paper presented to the American Public Health Association Annual Meeting on Oct. 21, 2001
Wellman, David, "Fast Track' Drug to Treat Diabetes Tied to 33 Deaths." Los Angeles Times, December 6, 1998
Wood, Alastair J.J. and others, "Making Medicines Safer -- The Need for an Independent Drug Safety Board," NEW ENGLAND JOURNAL OF MEDICINE Vol. 339, No. 25 (December 17, 1998), pgs. 1851-1854.
Journal of the American Medical Association ("Is a Gift Ever Just a Gift?", Vol. 283 No. 3, January 19, 2000)

Internet Reports

Adams, Mike. http://www.newstarget.com/ June 3, 2004, Mike Adams, "American Diabetes Association promotes statin drugs to diabetic patients without a shred of proof that they help"

FDA website http://www.fda.gov/bbs/topics/ANSWERS/2002/ANS01135.html

Graham, Dr. David, "Secrets of the FDA Revealed by Top Insider". (www.mercola.com/):

Null, Gary, PhD "Death By Medicine", http://www.nutritioninstituteofamerica.org/ (Click on "Research".)

USGAO, FDA DRUG REVIEW Postapproval Risks 1976-85. United States General Accounting Office (GAO) GAO/PEMD-90-15 Apr1990. p33

National Coalition on Health Care http://www.nchc.org/facts/cost.shtml